DIABETIC COOKBOOK MADE SIMPLE FOR SENIORS

1200+ Days of Easy and Delicious Recipes to Enhance Wellness, and Enjoy Flavorful Meals Every Day

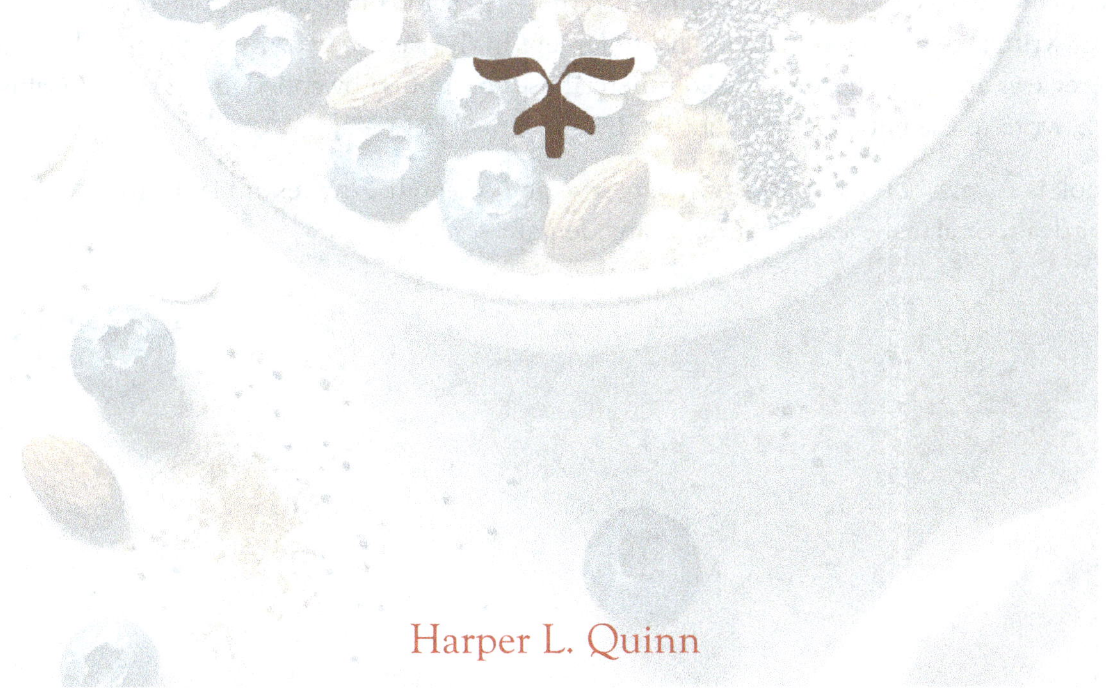

Harper L. Quinn

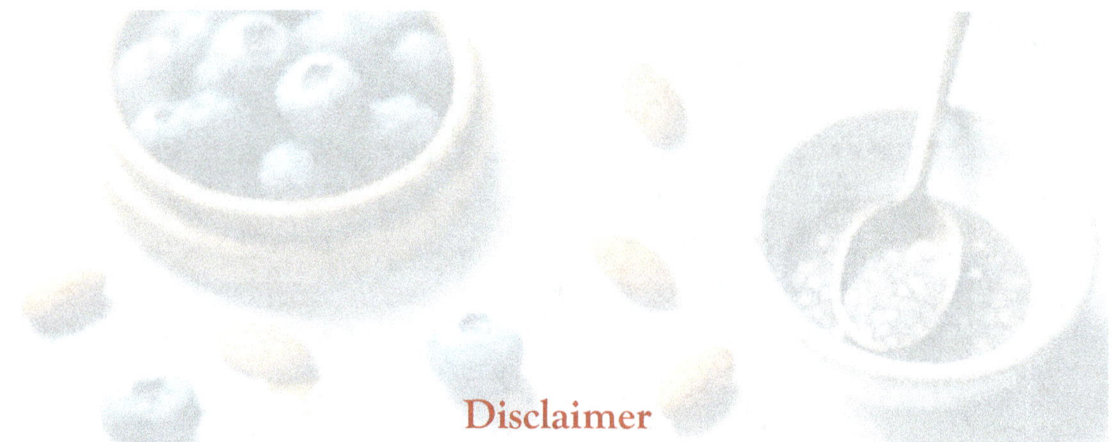

Disclaimer

The information contained in this cookbook is for educational and informational purposes only and is not intended as health or medical advice. The recipes and nutritional information provided are based on general guidelines for managing diabetes. Always consult with your physician or a qualified health professional before making any dietary changes, especially if you have any pre-existing medical conditions or concerns. The author and publisher are not responsible for any adverse effects or consequences resulting from the use of the recipes or suggestions in this book.

Copyright

Diabetic Cookbook Made Simple for Seniors

Contents

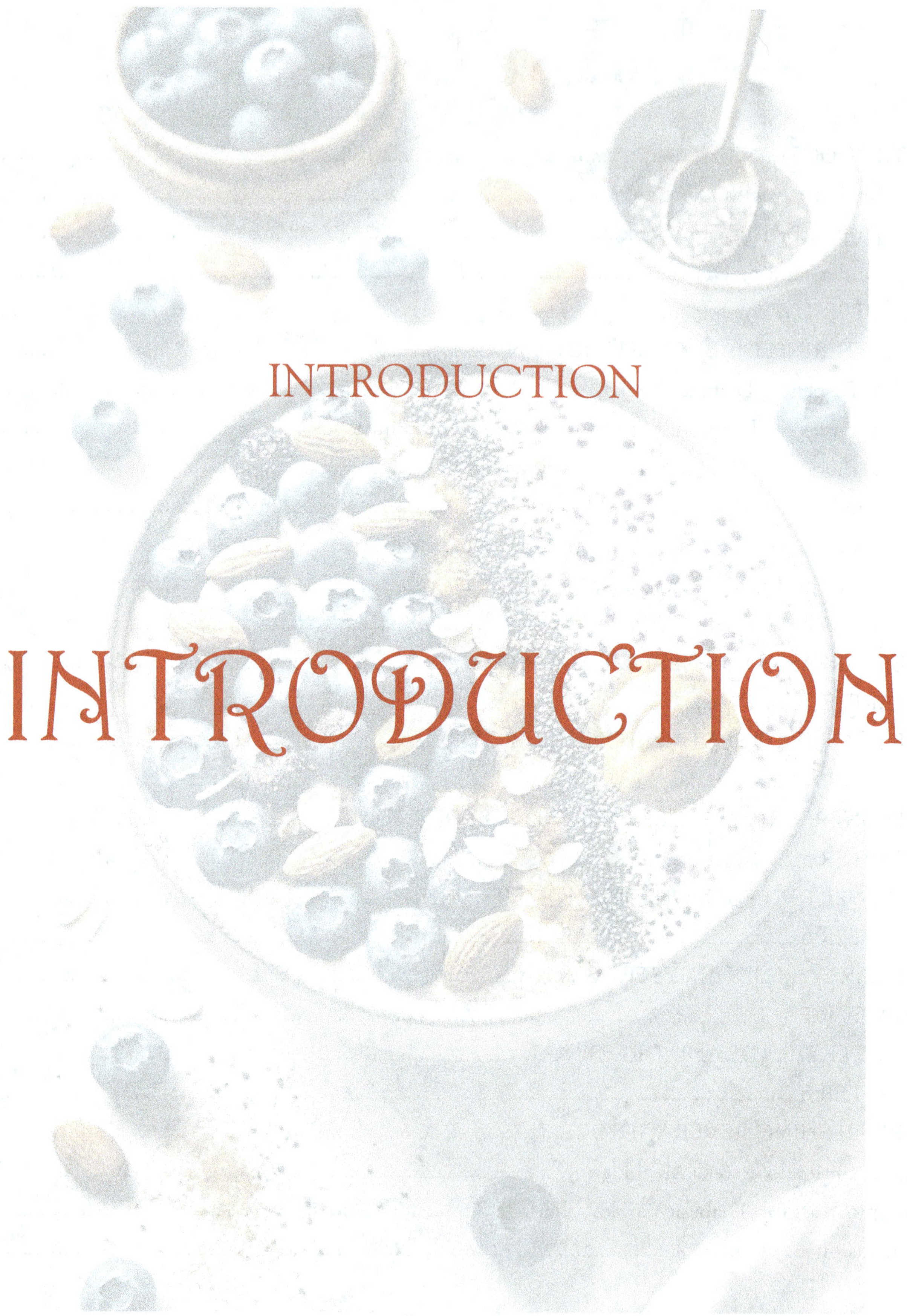

INTRODUCTION

INTRODUCTION

My Journey with Diabetes

Living with diabetes isn't just about managing numbers—it's about transforming your life. My journey began five years ago when I was diagnosed with Type 2 diabetes. The news hit me like a ton of bricks. I remember sitting in the doctor's office, feeling overwhelmed and uncertain about the future.

The initial shock soon gave way to determination. I knew I had to take control of my health, not just for myself but for my loved ones. The road was challenging, filled with trials and errors, but it also became a path of self-discovery and resilience. I learned to view food not just as a necessity but as a powerful tool for healing and nourishment.

One of my earliest challenges was rethinking my meals. I had always enjoyed hearty, comforting foods, and the idea of switching to a restrictive diet was daunting. But as I delved deeper into understanding diabetes and nutrition, I realized that healthy eating didn't mean giving up the flavors and dishes I loved. Instead, it was about finding creative and delicious ways to enjoy them.

This cookbook is the culmination of my journey, filled with recipes that are not only diabetes-friendly but also incredibly satisfying. Each recipe is a testament to the power of wholesome, nutritious food to transform our health and well-being.

As you embark on this culinary adventure, I hope you find joy, comfort, and inspiration in these dishes. Remember, managing diabetes is a marathon, not a sprint. Embrace the journey, savor each step, and know that you are not alone. Together, we can create a healthier, happier future.

Purpose of This Cookbook

"Diabetic Cookbook Made Simple for Seniors" – your new best friend in the kitchen! This isn't just any cookbook; it's your ticket to a world of delicious, diabetes-friendly meals that are as fun to make as they are to eat. We've ditched the boring, bland, and blah recipes and replaced them with vibrant, flavorful dishes that will have your taste buds dancing.

The goal here is simple: to make managing diabetes a delightful experience rather than a daunting task. Whether you're a seasoned cook or a kitchen newbie, you'll find these recipes easy to follow, quick to prepare, and packed with ingredients that love you back. No more guessing games about what to eat – we've got you covered from breakfast to dessert and everything in between.

So, put on your apron, grab your spatula, and let's whip up some magic in the kitchen. Because eating well with diabetes doesn't have to be a chore – it can be an adventure!

Understanding Diabetes

Ah, Diabetes – the uninvited guest that just won't leave! But fear not, with a little knowledge and a lot of delicious food, we can make this journey smoother.

Let's clear the fog and make understanding diabetes as simple as your morning coffee.

Diabetes is like a mischievous friend who constantly needs attention, especially when it comes to what you eat. It's all about balance: balancing your blood sugar levels, balancing your diet, and balancing your lifestyle. But don't worry, it's not rocket science – it's more like balancing on a seesaw. Once you get the hang of it, it becomes second nature.

Think of your body as a finely-tuned engine. With diabetes, you just need to be a bit more mindful of the fuel you put in. Carbs, proteins, and fats all play a role in how your body runs, and understanding this interplay is key. Too many carbs, and your blood sugar spikes like a caffeine rush. Too few, and you might feel like a deflated balloon.

But here's the kicker: managing diabetes doesn't mean giving up the foods you love. It's about making smarter choices, finding delicious alternatives, and sometimes indulging in a guilt-free treat. After all, life is too short for boring food.

So, let's embrace this journey with a sprinkle of humor and a dash of determination. Together, we can navigate the ups and downs of diabetes with confidence and a smile. Remember, managing diabetes is not about restriction – it's about empowerment and enjoying every bite along the way!

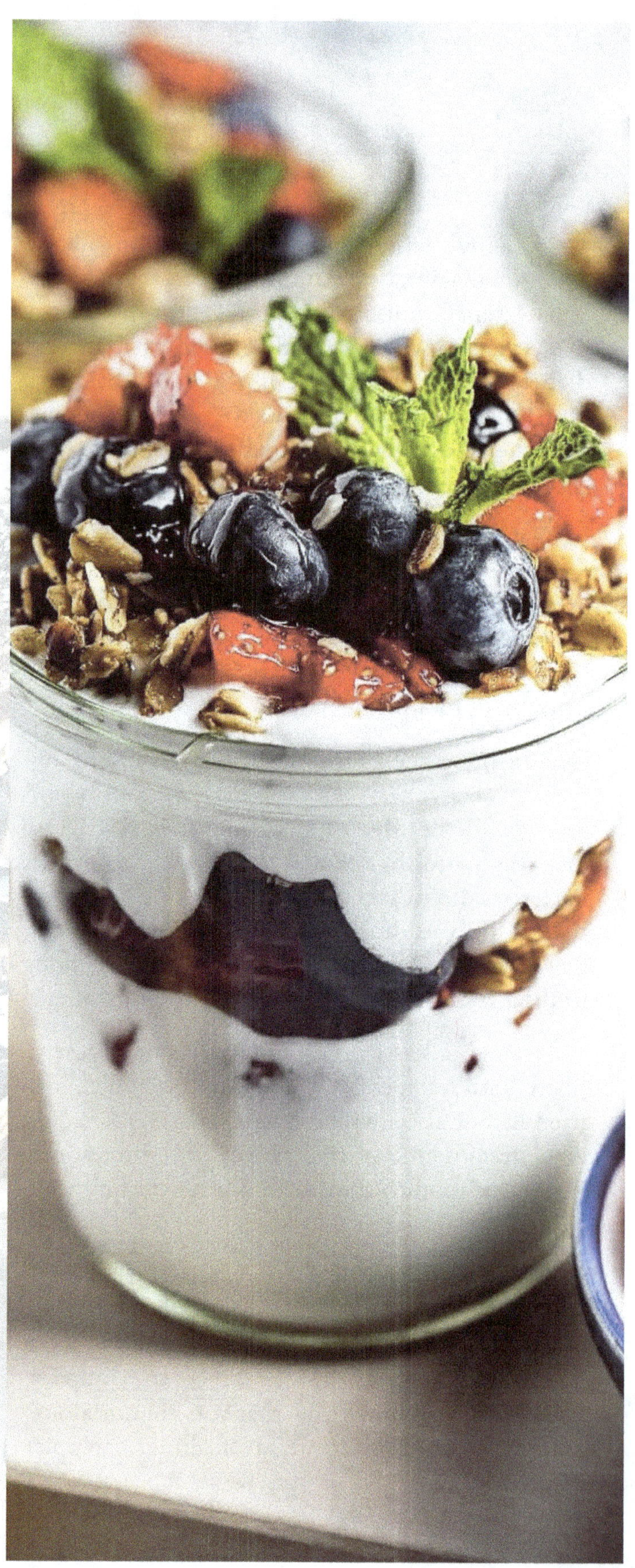

CHAPTER 1

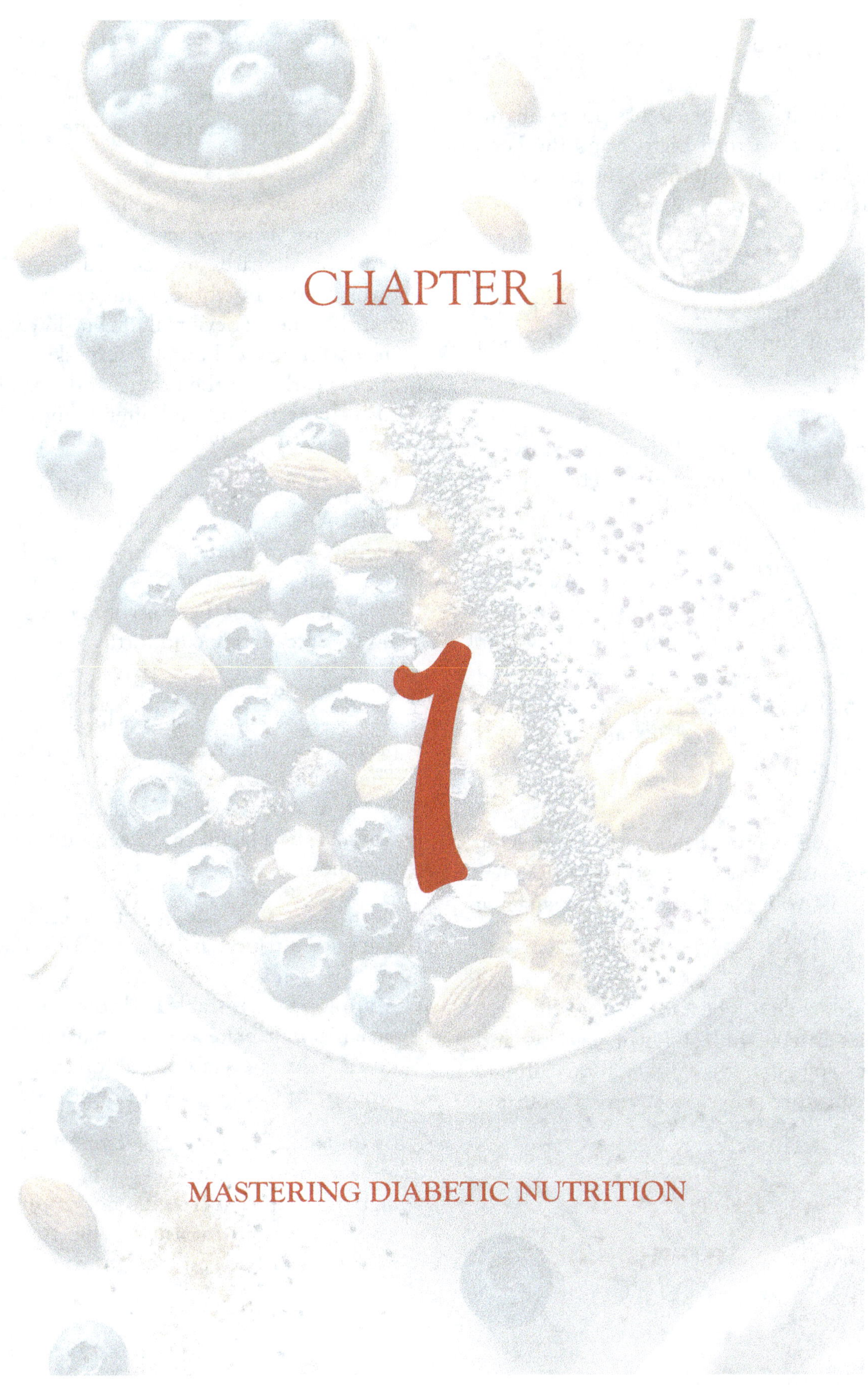

MASTERING DIABETIC NUTRITION

1. Dispelling Diabetes Myths

Let's face it – diabetes has more myths surrounding it than Bigfoot and the Loch Ness Monster combined. Let us set the record straight, one myth at a time.

Myth #1: Diabetics Can Never Eat Sugar False! While it's important to monitor your sugar intake, the occasional treat won't send your health spiraling out of control. The key is moderation and balance.

Myth #2: Carbs Are the Enemy Wrong again! Carbohydrates are not the villain of this story. In fact, they're essential for energy. The trick is choosing the right carbs – think whole grains, vegetables, and legumes – and avoiding those sneaky refined sugars.

Myth #3: Only Overweight People Get Diabetes Nope! Diabetes doesn't discriminate. While being overweight can increase your risk, genetics and other factors play a significant role. So, if someone gives you unsolicited diet advice, just smile and know the truth.

Myth #4: You Can Feel When Your Blood Sugar is High or Low Sometimes you might, but relying on "feeling" isn't the best strategy. Regular monitoring is your best friend in managing diabetes effectively.

Myth #5: Diabetics Can Only Eat Bland Food Let's put this one to bed forever. A diabetic-friendly diet can be full of flavor, variety, and excitement. Spices, herbs, and a little culinary creativity can turn any meal into a gourmet experience.

2. Basics of Nutrition: Macronutrients and Their Impact

Now that we've busted those myths, let's dive into the nitty-gritty of nutrition. It's time to get to know your macronutrients – the big three that make up your diet: carbohydrates, proteins, and fats.

Carbohydrates: Carbs are like the fuel in your car – they give you the energy to get through the day. But not all carbs are created equal. Complex carbs, found in whole grains and vegetables, are your best bet. They break down slowly, providing steady energy without those pesky sugar spikes. Simple carbs, on the other hand, are like a sugar rush – fast, fleeting, and often followed by a crash. Choose wisely.

Proteins: Proteins are the building blocks of your body. They help repair tissues, build muscle, and keep your immune system strong. Lean meats, fish, beans, and nuts are excellent sources of protein. Think of them as your body's repair crew, always on call to fix and fortify.

Fats: Fats often get a bad rap, but they're essential for your health. They help absorb vitamins, protect your organs, and keep your skin glowing. The trick is to focus on healthy fats like those found in avocados, nuts, and olive oil. Avoid trans fats like the plague, and keep saturated fats to a minimum.

Balancing Act: The secret sauce to mastering diabetic nutrition is balance. Each meal should include a mix of these macronutrients to keep your blood sugar stable and your energy levels up. Imagine your plate as a pie chart: half filled with non-starchy vegetables, a quarter with lean protein, and a quarter with healthy carbs.

By understanding these macronutrients and their impact on your body, you can take control of your diet and your diabetes. It's not about restriction; it's about making informed, delicious choices that nourish your body and delight your taste buds.

3. Blood Sugar Monitoring: Techniques and Tips

Monitoring your blood sugar is like having a GPS for your diabetes management – it guides you, keeps you on the right path, and helps you avoid unexpected detours. Let's explore the essentials of blood sugar monitoring, backed by research and sprinkled with a dash of wit.

Why Monitor Your Blood Sugar? Monitoring your blood sugar levels isn't just for show – it's a crucial part of managing diabetes. By keeping tabs on your glucose levels, you can:

- **Make informed decisions** about your diet, exercise, and medications.

- **Prevent complications** such as nerve damage, kidney disease, and vision problems.

- **Stay on track** with your health goals and enjoy a better quality of life.

When to Monitor: Timing is everything. Here's a quick rundown of the key times to check your blood sugar:

- **Fasting:** First thing in the morning, before you've had anything to eat or drink.

- **Before meals:** To gauge your baseline levels.

- **Two hours after meals:** To see how your body is handling the food.

- **Before and after exercise:** Physical activity can lower blood sugar, so it's good to know where you stand.

- **Before bedtime:** To ensure your levels are stable before sleep.

- **Whenever you feel "off":** If you're feeling unusually tired, shaky, or irritable, it's a good idea to check.

Tools of the Trade: Let's talk gadgets. Here are the essentials for blood sugar monitoring:

- **Glucometer:** The classic choice. It's reliable, portable, and gives you results in seconds.

- **Continuous Glucose Monitor (CGM):** For those who like a high-tech approach. A CGM provides real-time data and trends by measuring glucose in the interstitial fluid every few minutes. Perfect for the tech-savvy senior.

- **Test Strips and Lancets:** These are the sidekicks to your glucometer. Test strips analyze the blood sample, while lancets provide a quick (and relatively painless) poke.

Technique Tips: Getting an accurate reading is more than just a finger prick. Here's how to do it right:

- **Wash your hands:** Clean hands prevent contamination and ensure accurate readings. No one wants chocolate cake residue skewing the results!

- **Use the sides of your fingers:** The sides are less sensitive than the pads, making the process more comfortable.

- **Rotate fingers:** Avoid overusing one finger to prevent soreness and calluses.

- **Stay relaxed:** Stress can affect your blood sugar levels. Take a few deep breaths and stay calm before testing.

Logging Your Results: Keep a record of your readings. It's like maintaining a diary for your blood sugar levels. You can use:

- **A notebook:** Classic and simple.

- **Apps:** Many apps sync with your glucometer or CGM, making tracking a breeze.

- **Charts or spreadsheets**: For the data enthusiasts who love seeing patterns and trends.

Making Sense of the Numbers: Here's where the fun begins – interpreting your readings. Here are some general guidelines:

- **Fasting Blood Sugar**: Aim for 80-130 mg/dL.

- **Two Hours after Meals**: Ideally, it should be below 180 mg/dL.

- **Individual Targets**: Your doctor may set personalized targets based on your overall health and diabetes management plan.

Problem Solving: What if your numbers are off? Don't panic. Here's what you can do:

- **High readings**: Review your recent meals, exercise, and stress levels. Adjust your diet, take a walk, or follow your doctor's advice for medication.

- **Low readings**: Have a quick snack with carbs (like fruit juice or glucose tablets). Recheck after 15 minutes to ensure it's rising.

Monitoring your blood sugar doesn't have to be a chore. With the right techniques and tools, it becomes a straightforward part of your daily routine, empowering you to live your best life with diabetes.

Foods to Avoid and Foods to Eat

Managing diabetes effectively hinges on understanding which foods to embrace and which to avoid. Let's delve into this with a professional yet approachable lens, backed by research and practical experience.

Foods to Avoid

1. **Sugary Beverages**

   o **Why Avoid:** These are loaded with simple sugars that cause rapid spikes in blood glucose levels.

   o **Examples:** Soda, fruit juices, sweetened teas, and energy drinks.

   o **Research Insight:** A study in the *Journal of the American Medical Association* found that sugary beverages significantly increase the risk of type 2 diabetes.

2. **Trans Fats**

   o **Why Avoid:** Trans fats are linked to inflammation, insulin resistance, and increased belly fat.

   o **Examples:** Partially hydrogenated oils found in margarine, packaged baked goods, and fried fast food.

   o **Research Insight:** The *American Heart Association* advises eliminating trans-fats from your diet due to their adverse effects on heart health and blood sugar control.

3. **Refined Carbohydrates**

   o **Why Avoid:** These carbs are stripped of fiber and nutrients, leading to quick blood sugar spikes.

   o **Examples:** White bread, white rice, pasta, and pastries.

   o **Research Insight:** According to a study published in *The Lancet*, diets high in refined carbs are associated with a higher risk of type 2 diabetes.

4. **Processed Meats**

   o **Why Avoid:** High in sodium and preservatives, processed meats can increase the risk of heart disease and diabetes complications.

   o **Examples:** Bacon, sausages, hot dogs, and deli meats.

   o **Research Insight:** The *Harvard School of Public Health* reports that regular consumption of processed meats is linked to a 42% higher risk of heart disease and a 19% higher risk of diabetes.

5. **Sugary Cereals**

   o **Why Avoid:** These cereals often contain high amounts of added sugars and lack essential nutrients.

   o **Examples:** Many brands of breakfast cereals marketed to children and adults alike.

   o **Research Insight:** A study in *Diabetes Care* found that high sugar intake from cereals correlates with poorer blood sugar control .

Foods to Eat

1. **Non-Starchy Vegetables**

   o **Why Eat:** Packed with fiber, vitamins, and minerals, they help manage blood sugar levels and support overall health.

   o **Examples:** Spinach, broccoli, peppers, and cucumbers.

   o **Research Insight:** The *American Diabetes Association* recommends filling half your plate with non-starchy vegetables at each meal to help control blood sugar.

2. **Whole Grains**

   o **Why Eat:** Rich in fiber and nutrients, whole grains have a lower glycemic index and promote gradual blood sugar rise.

   o **Examples:** Brown rice, quinoa, oatmeal, and whole-wheat bread.

   o **Research Insight:** A study in *The Journal of Nutrition* found that whole grain consumption is associated with a reduced risk of type 2 diabetes and better glycemic control.

3. **Lean Proteins**

   o **Why Eat:** Protein helps with satiety and blood sugar management without spiking glucose levels.

   o **Examples:** Chicken breast, turkey, fish, tofu, and legumes.

   o **Research Insight:** According to the *American Journal of Clinical Nutrition*, high-protein diets can improve blood glucose stability and aid in weight management.

4. **Healthy Fats**

   o **Why Eat:** Healthy fats support heart health and can improve insulin sensitivity.

   o **Examples:** Avocados, nuts, seeds, and olive oil.

   o **Research Insight:** The *British Medical Journal* published findings that diets rich in monounsaturated and polyunsaturated fats are beneficial for glycemic control and cardiovascular health.

5. **Berries and Citrus Fruits**

   o **Why Eat:** These fruits are high in fiber, vitamins, and antioxidants, and have a lower glycemic impact.

   o **Examples:** Strawberries, blueberries, oranges, and grapefruits.

   o **Research Insight:** A study in *Nutrition Research* highlighted that moderate fruit intake is associated with better glycemic control and reduced diabetes complications .

By focusing on these dietary choices, you can effectively manage your diabetes while enjoying a diverse and flavorful diet. Remember, it's not just about avoiding certain foods but also about embracing those that nourish and support your health.

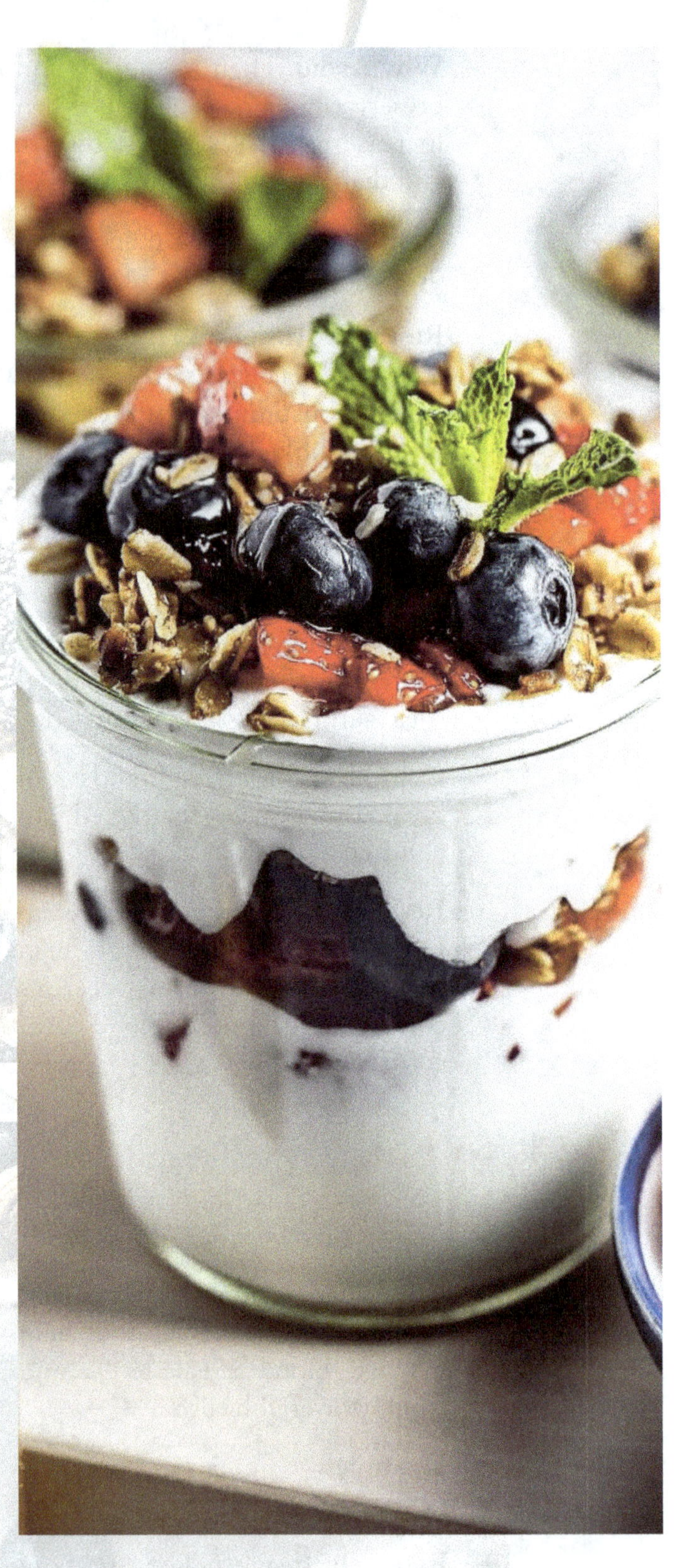

CHAPTER 2

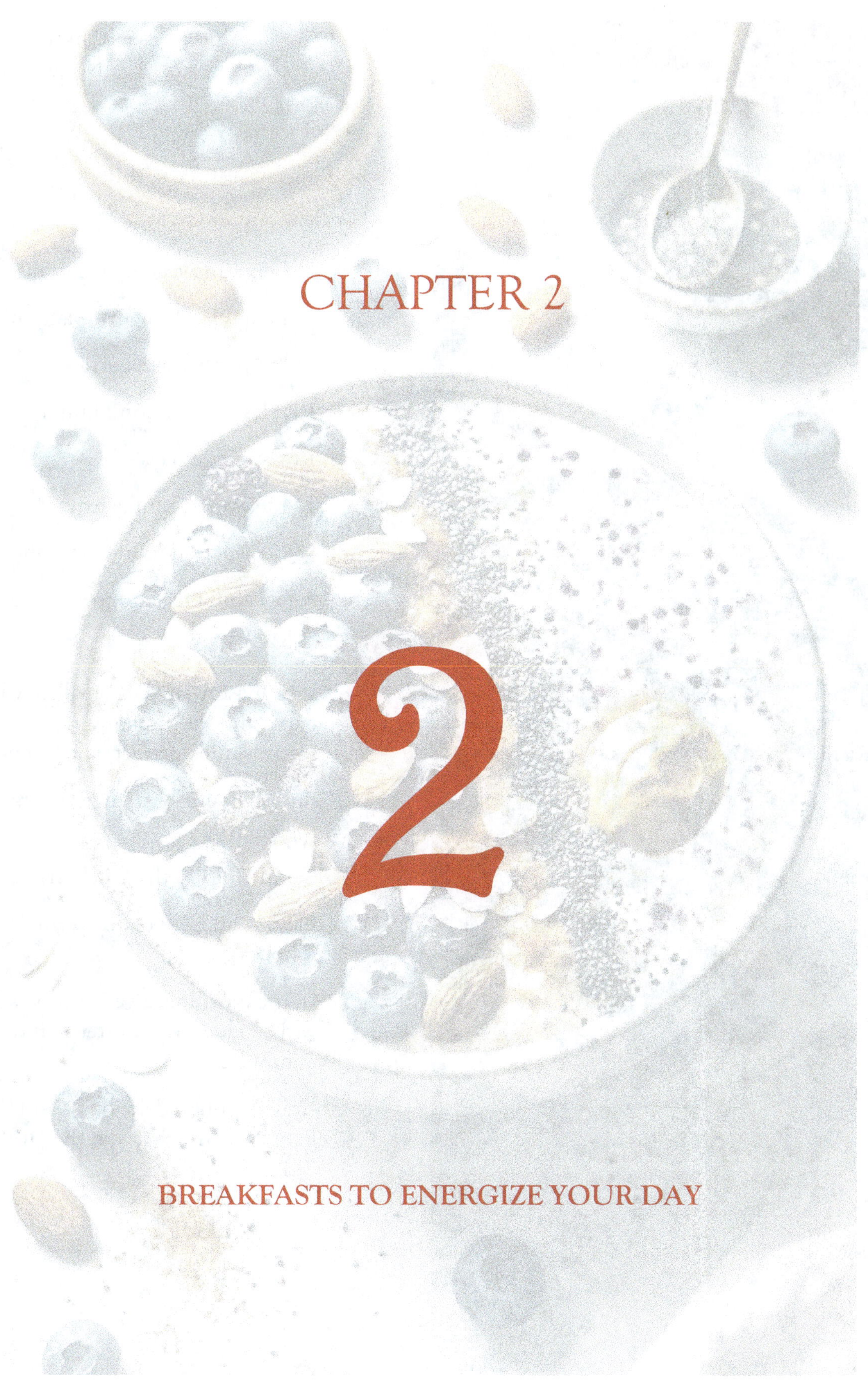

2

BREAKFASTS TO ENERGIZE YOUR DAY

Blueberry Almond Overnight Oats

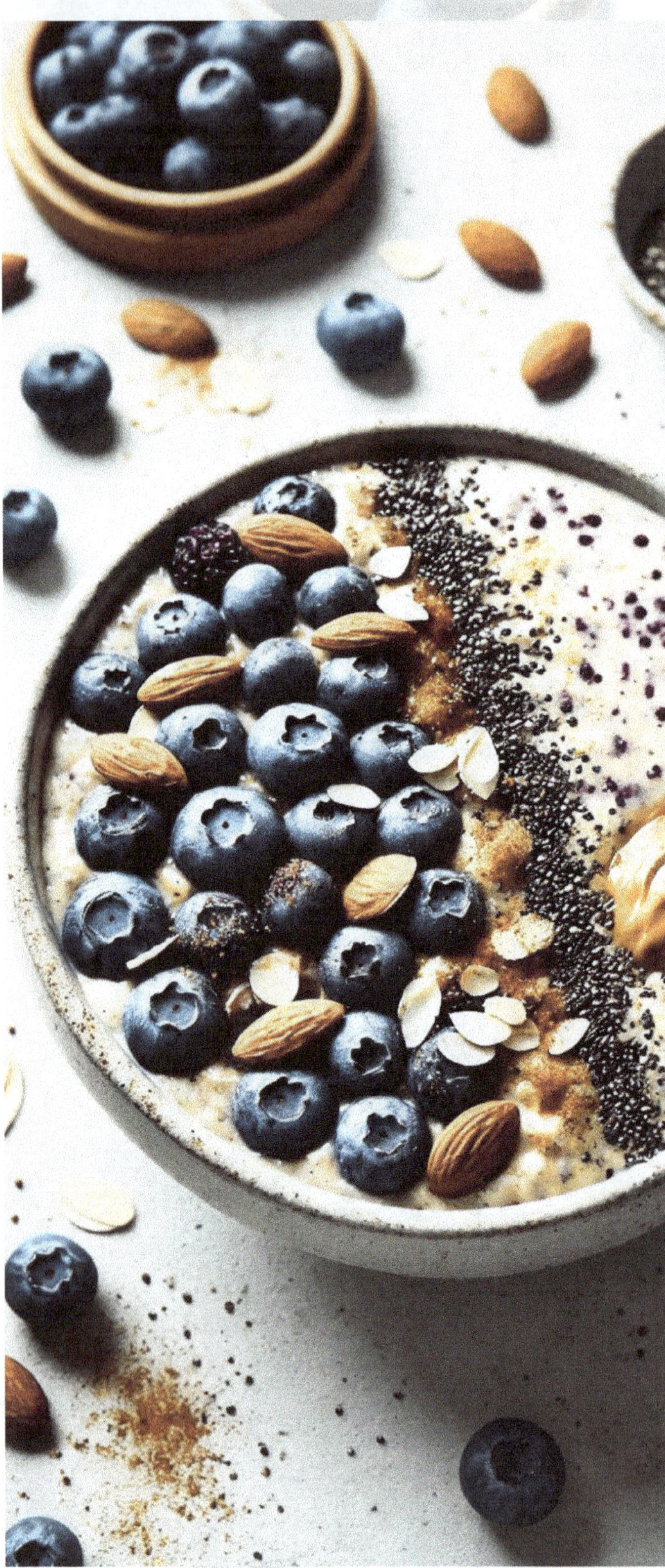

- **Preparation Time:** 10 minutes
- **Cooking Time:** None (Refrigerate overnight)
- **Serving:** 1

Ingredients:

- 1/2 cup old-fashioned rolled oats
- 1/2 cup unsweetened almond milk
- 1/4 cup Greek yogurt (plain, non-fat)
- 1/4 cup fresh blueberries
- 1 tablespoon almond butter
- 1 teaspoon chia seeds
- 1/4 teaspoon vanilla extract
- 1/4 teaspoon ground cinnamon
- A few almonds, chopped (for garnish)

Procedure:

1. In a mason jar or a small bowl, combine oats, almond milk, Greek yogurt, chia seeds, vanilla extract, and cinnamon.
2. Stir well until all ingredients are mixed together.
3. Gently fold in the blueberries.
4. Cover and refrigerate overnight (or at least 4 hours).
5. In the morning, give it a good stir, and top with almond butter and chopped almonds.
6. Enjoy your delicious and nutritious breakfast straight from the jar or bowl.

Nutritional Values (per serving):

- Calories: 250
- Protein: 10g
- Carbohydrates: 32g

- Fiber: 7g

- Sugars: 8g

- Fat: 9g

- Saturated Fat: 1g

- Sodium: 95mg

Health Benefits:

- The combination of oats and chia seeds provides a steady release of energy, helping to maintain stable blood sugar levels.

- Almonds and almond milk offer healthy fats that support heart health.

- High in fiber, this recipe promotes good digestion and keeps you feeling full longer.

Spinach and Feta Egg Muffins

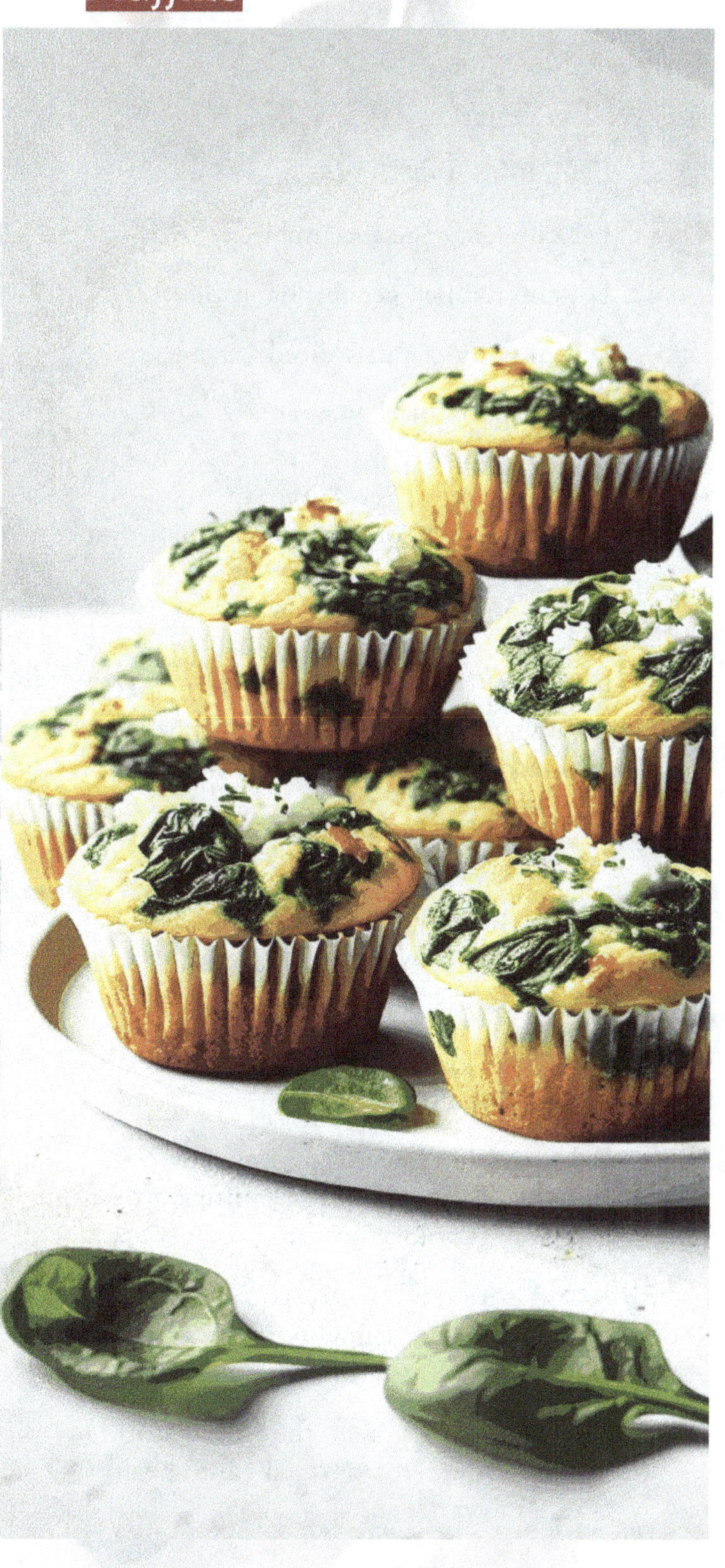

- **Preparation Time:** 10 minutes
- **Cooking Time:** 20 minutes
- **Serving:** 6 muffins

Ingredients:

- 6 large eggs
- 1 cup fresh spinach, chopped
- 1/2 cup feta cheese, crumbled
- 1/4 cup red bell pepper, finely diced
- 1/4 cup onion, finely diced
- 1/4 teaspoon black pepper
- 1/4 teaspoon salt
- Cooking spray or a little olive oil for greasing

Procedure:

1. Preheat your oven to 350°F (175°C). Lightly grease a 6-cup muffin tin with cooking spray or olive oil.

2. In a large bowl, whisk together the eggs, salt, and pepper.

3. Stir in the chopped spinach, feta cheese, red bell pepper, and onion until well combined.

4. Pour the egg mixture evenly into the prepared muffin cups.

5. Bake in the preheated oven for 18-20 minutes, or until the egg muffins are set and slightly golden on top.

6. Allow the muffins to cool for a few minutes before removing them from the tin.

7. Enjoy warm, or store in the refrigerator for up to 3 days for a quick and healthy breakfast on the go.

Nutritional Values (per muffin):

- Calories: 70
- Protein: 6g
- Carbohydrates: 2g
- Fiber: 0.5g
- Sugars: 1g
- Fat: 4g
- Saturated Fat: 2g
- Sodium: 200mg

Health Benefits:

- **Protein-Packed:** Eggs provide high-quality protein that helps in maintaining muscle mass and keeping you satiated.

- **Rich in Vitamins:** Spinach offers a good dose of vitamins A, C, and K, along with iron and calcium.

- **Low-Glycemic:** These muffins are low in carbohydrates, making them ideal for managing blood sugar levels.

Cinnamon Apple Quinoa Bowl

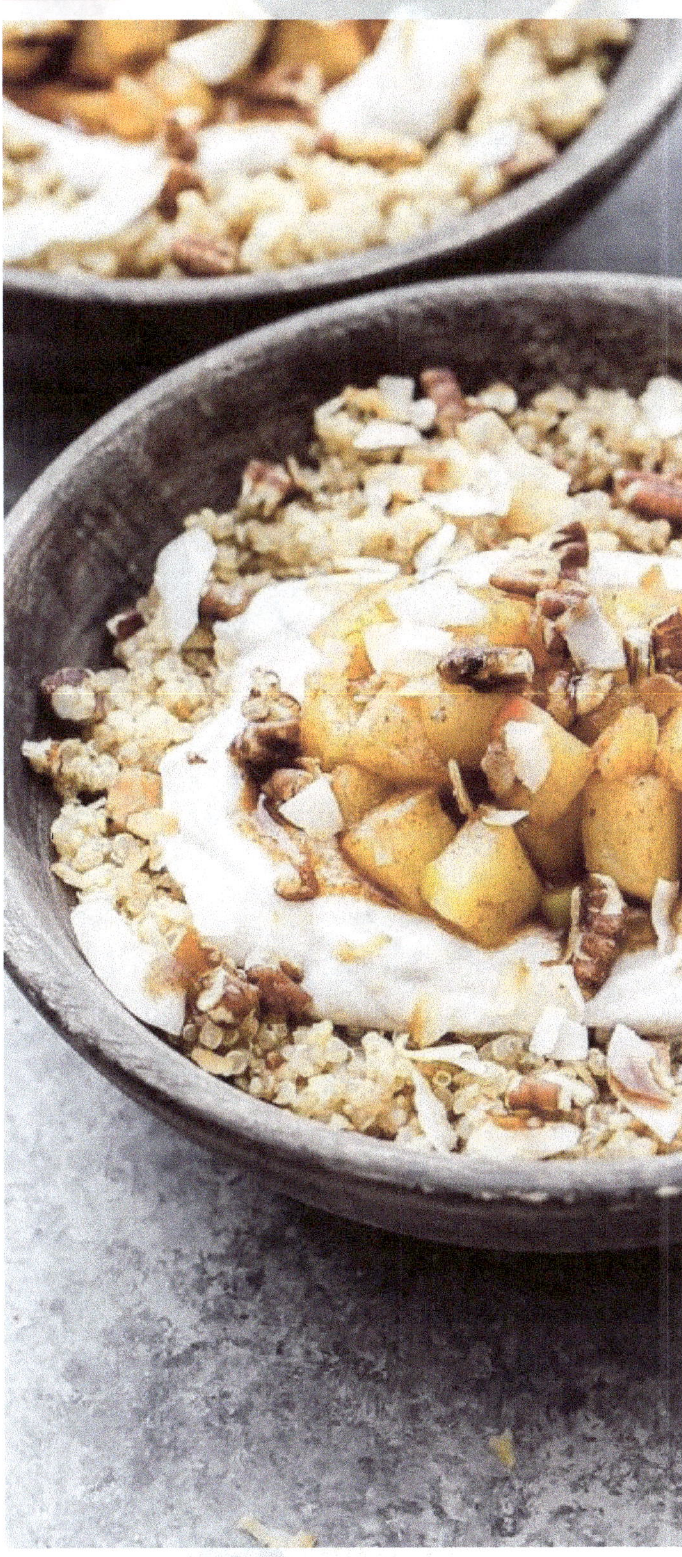

- **Preparation Time:** 10 minutes
- **Cooking Time:** 20 minutes
- **Serving:** 2

Ingredients:

- 1/2 cup quinoa
- 1 cup water
- 1 medium apple, diced
- 1/2 teaspoon ground cinnamon
- 1/4 teaspoon ground nutmeg
- 1 tablespoon chia seeds
- 1/4 cup unsweetened almond milk
- 1 tablespoon chopped walnuts
- 1 tablespoon raisins (optional)
- A pinch of salt

Procedure:

1. Rinse quinoa under cold water to remove any bitterness.
2. In a small saucepan, combine quinoa and water. Bring to a boil over medium heat.
3. Reduce heat to low, cover, and simmer for about 15 minutes or until quinoa is tender and water is absorbed.
4. While the quinoa is cooking, dice the apple.
5. Once the quinoa is done, stir in the diced apple, cinnamon, nutmeg, chia seeds, and a pinch of salt.
6. Cook for an additional 5 minutes, stirring occasionally until the apples are tender.
7. Remove from heat and stir in the almond milk.
8. Divide the quinoa mixture into two bowls.

9. Top with chopped walnuts and raisins, if using.

10. Serve warm and enjoy!

Nutritional Values (per serving):

- Calories: 250

- Protein: 6g

- Carbohydrates: 40g

- Fiber: 6g

- Sugars: 10g

- Fat: 8g

- Saturated Fat: 1g

- Sodium: 50mg

Health Benefits:

- **Blood Sugar Management:** Quinoa is a low-glycemic grain that helps keep blood sugar levels stable.

- **Heart Health:** Walnuts and chia seeds provide healthy fats that support cardiovascular health.

- **High Fiber:** Apples and quinoa offer a good amount of fiber, aiding digestion and keeping you full longer.

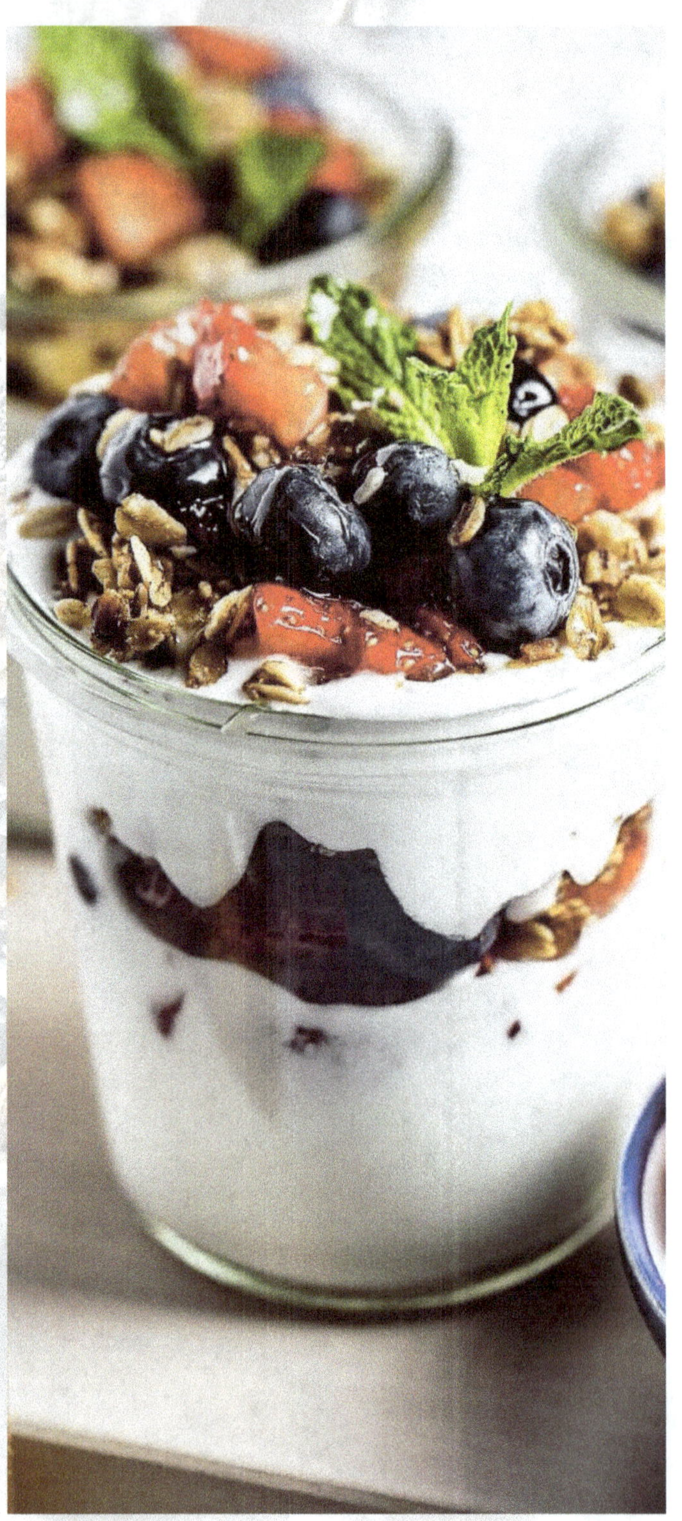

Greek Yogurt Parfait with Berries and Nuts

- **Preparation Time:** 5 minutes
- **Cooking Time:** None
- **Serving:** 1

Ingredients:

- 1 cup plain Greek yogurt (non-fat or low-fat)
- 1/2 cup mixed berries (blueberries, strawberries, raspberries)
- 1 tablespoon chopped almonds
- 1 tablespoon chia seeds
- 1 teaspoon honey or a few drops of stevia (optional)

Procedure:

1. In a serving glass or bowl, layer half of the Greek yogurt.
2. Add half of the mixed berries on top of the yogurt layer.
3. Sprinkle half of the chopped almonds and chia seeds over the berries.
4. Repeat the layers with the remaining yogurt, berries, almonds, and chia seeds.
5. Drizzle with honey or stevia, if desired.
6. Serve immediately and enjoy!

Nutritional Values (per serving):

- Calories: 200
- Protein: 15g
- Carbohydrates: 20g
- Fiber: 6g
- Sugars: 12g (natural sugars from berries)
- Fat: 7g
- Saturated Fat: 1g
- Sodium: 60mg

Health Benefits:

- **High Protein:** Greek yogurt provides a substantial amount of protein, helping to maintain muscle mass and keeping you full.
- **Antioxidants:** Berries are rich in antioxidants, which help combat inflammation and support overall health.
- **Healthy Fats:** Almonds and chia seeds offer healthy fats that aid in blood sugar management and heart health.

Veggie-Packed Breakfast Burrito

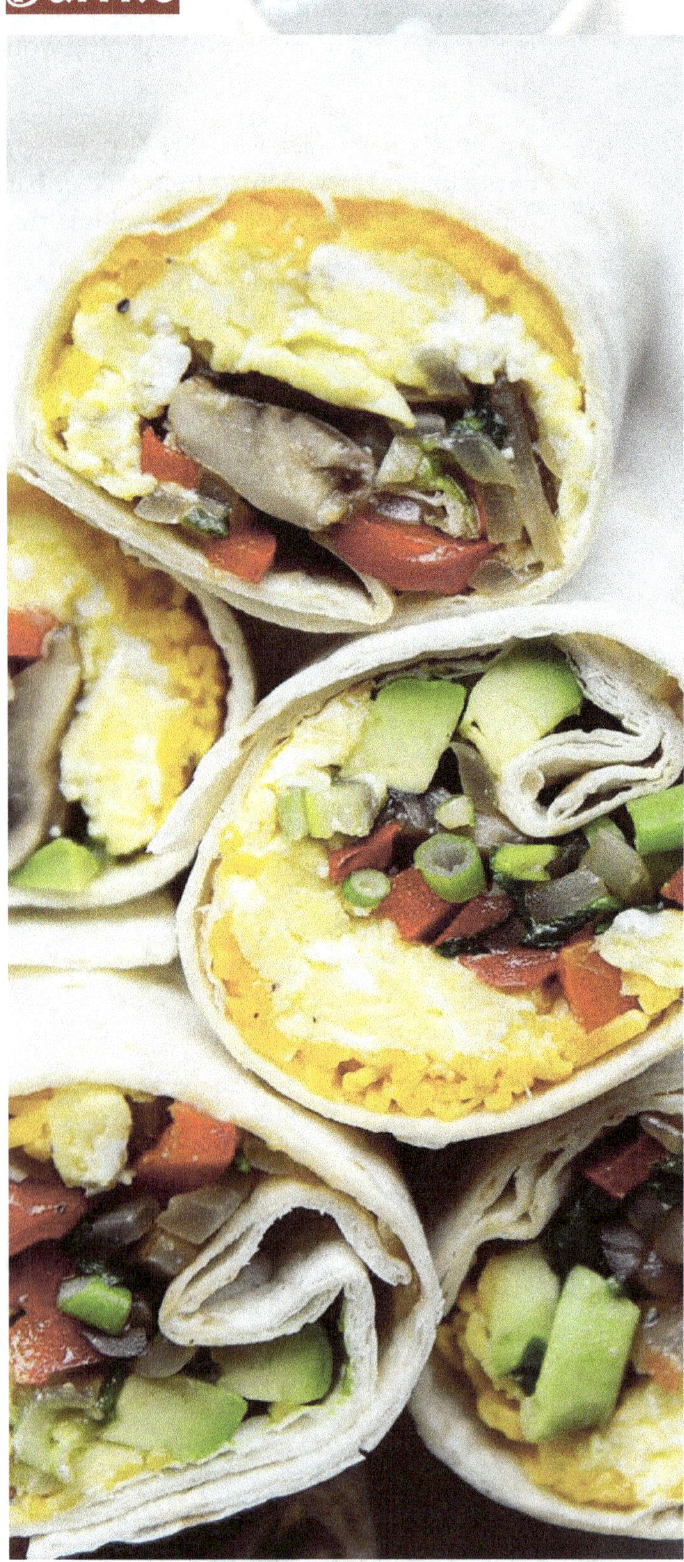

- Preparation Time: 10 minutes
- Cooking Time: 10 minutes
- Serving: 1

Ingredients:

- 1 whole grain tortilla
- 2 large eggs
- 1/4 cup bell pepper, diced (red or green)
- 1/4 cup spinach, chopped
- 1/4 cup mushrooms, sliced
- 1/4 avocado, sliced
- 1 tablespoon shredded low-fat cheese (optional)
- 1 tablespoon salsa (optional)
- 1/4 teaspoon black pepper
- 1/4 teaspoon salt
- 1 teaspoon olive oil

Procedure:

1. In a small bowl, whisk the eggs with a pinch of salt and pepper.
2. Heat the olive oil in a non-stick skillet over medium heat.
3. Add the bell pepper, spinach, and mushrooms to the skillet. Sauté for about 3-4 minutes until vegetables are tender.
4. Pour the whisked eggs into the skillet and cook, stirring occasionally, until the eggs are scrambled and fully cooked.
5. Warm the whole grain tortilla in a separate skillet or microwave for about 20 seconds until pliable.
6. Place the scrambled eggs and veggie mixture onto the center of the tortilla.

7. Add the avocado slices on top, followed by shredded cheese and salsa, if using.

8. Roll up the tortilla, folding in the sides, and enjoy your veggie-packed breakfast burrito.

Nutritional Values (per serving):

- Calories: 300

- Protein: 14g

- Carbohydrates: 25g

- Fiber: 8g

- Sugars: 3g

- Fat: 17g

- Saturated Fat: 4g

- Sodium: 450mg

Health Benefits:

- **High Fiber:** Whole grain tortilla and vegetables provide fiber that helps manage blood sugar levels and promotes digestive health.

- **Healthy Fats:** Avocado and olive oil offer heart-healthy monounsaturated fats.

- **Protein-Packed:** Eggs provide high-quality protein, essential for muscle maintenance and satiety.

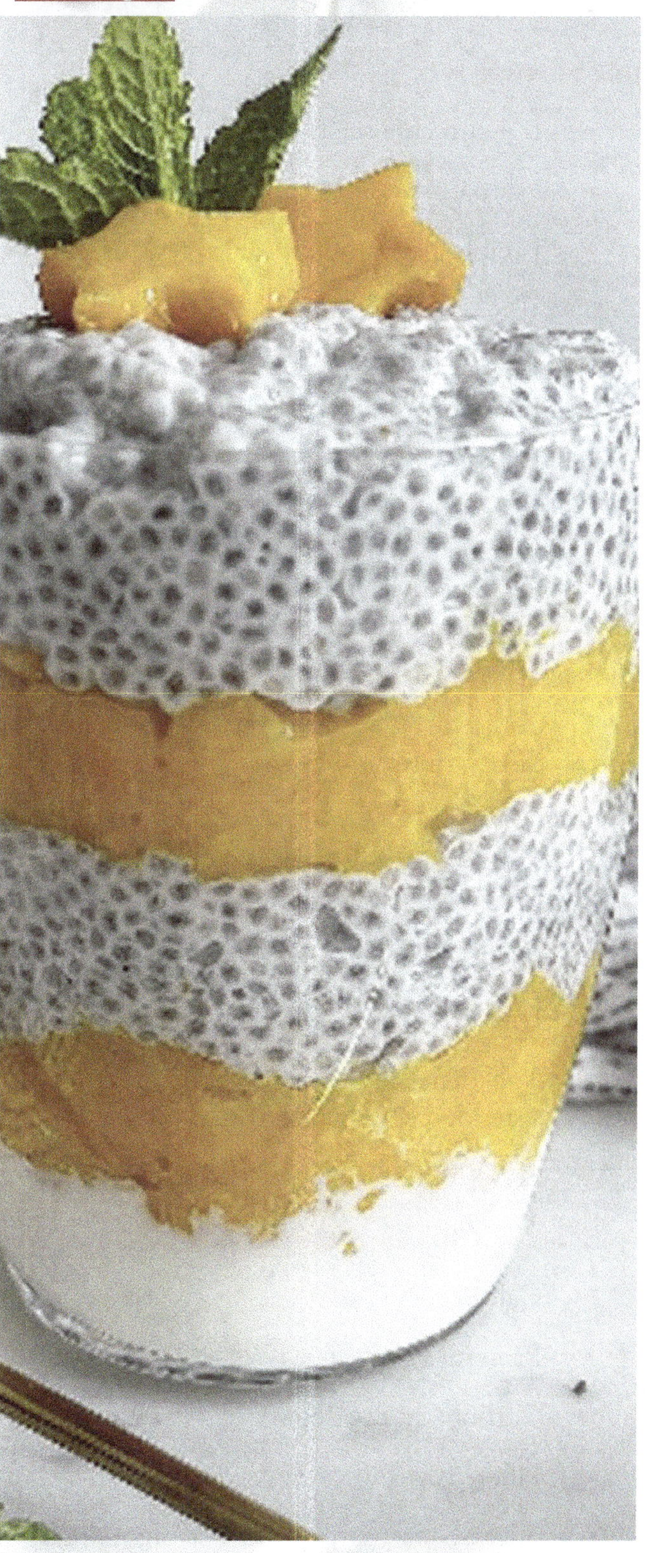

Chia Seed Pudding with Mango

- **Preparation Time:** 10 minutes
- **Cooking Time:** None (Refrigerate overnight)
- **Serving:** 2

Ingredients:

- 1/4 cup chia seeds
- 1 cup unsweetened almond milk
- 1 tablespoon honey or a few drops of stevia (optional)
- 1/2 teaspoon vanilla extract
- 1/2 cup fresh mango, diced
- 1 tablespoon shredded coconut (optional)

Procedure:

1. In a medium bowl, combine chia seeds, almond milk, honey or stevia, and vanilla extract.
2. Stir well to ensure chia seeds are evenly distributed.
3. Cover the bowl and refrigerate overnight or for at least 4 hours.
4. Once the pudding has set, stir again to break up any clumps.
5. Divide the chia pudding into two servings.
6. Top each serving with diced mango and shredded coconut, if using.
7. Serve immediately and enjoy!

Nutritional Values (per serving):

- Calories: 200
- Protein: 5g
- Carbohydrates: 28g
- Fiber: 10g
- Sugars: 15g (natural sugars from mango)
- Fat: 9g
- Saturated Fat: 2g
- Sodium: 50mg

Health Benefits:

- **Blood Sugar Management:** Chia seeds are low-glycemic and help stabilize blood sugar levels.
- **Rich in Omega-3:** Chia seeds provide essential omega-3 fatty acids, promoting heart health.
- **High Fiber:** Both chia seeds and mango contribute to a high fiber content, aiding digestion and satiety.

Whole Grain Avocado Toast

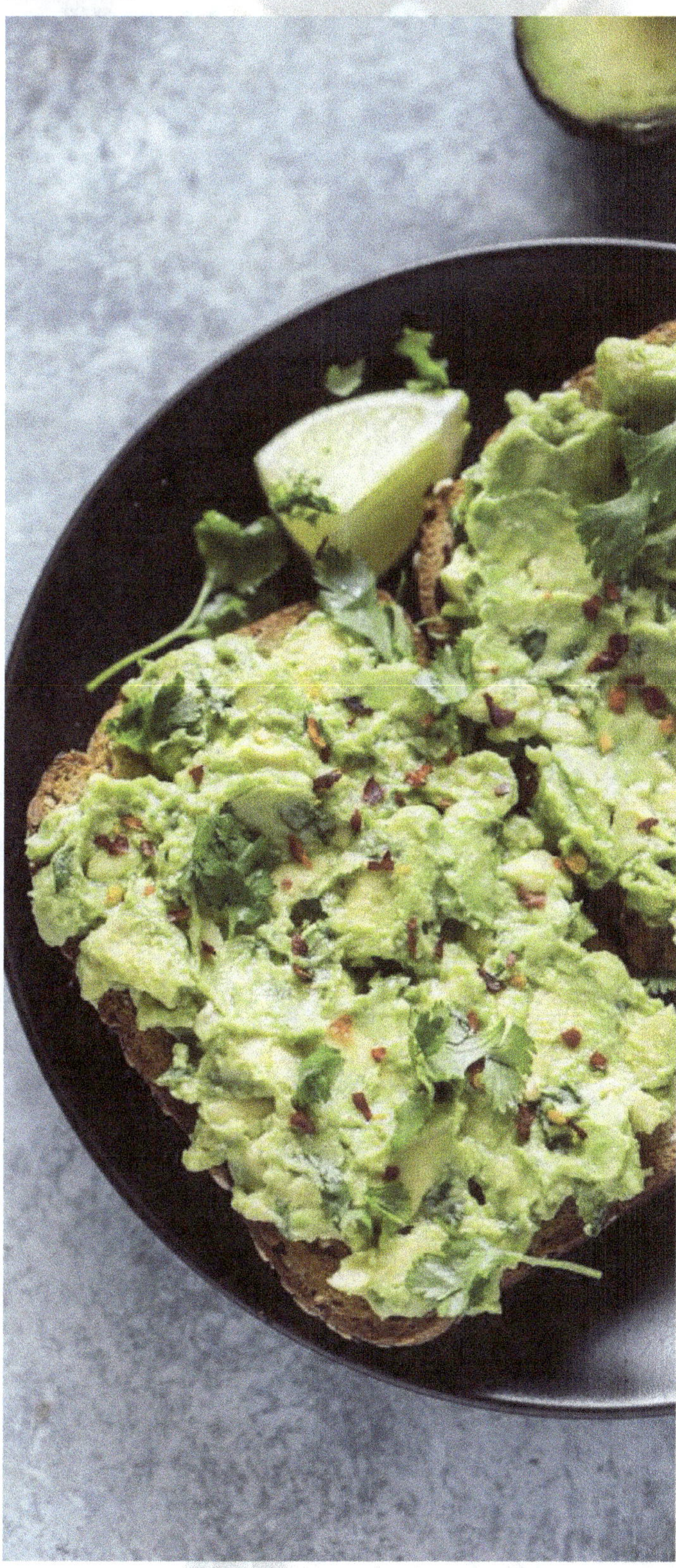

- **Preparation Time:** 5 minutes
- **Cooking Time:** 5 minutes
- **Serving:** 1

Ingredients:

- 1 slice whole grain bread
- 1/2 ripe avocado
- 1/4 teaspoon black pepper
- 1/4 teaspoon red pepper flakes (optional)
- 1 teaspoon lemon juice
- 1/4 teaspoon sea salt
- 1 small radish, thinly sliced (optional)

Procedure:

1. Toast the whole grain bread until golden and crisp.
2. While the bread is toasting, scoop out the avocado into a small bowl.
3. Mash the avocado with a fork until smooth.
4. Mix in the lemon juice, sea salt, and black pepper.
5. Spread the mashed avocado evenly over the toasted bread.
6. Sprinkle red pepper flakes on top for a bit of heat, if desired.
7. Add thinly sliced radish on top for extra crunch, if using.
8. Serve immediately and enjoy!

Nutritional Values (per serving):

- Calories: 250
- Protein: 6g
- Carbohydrates: 28g
- Fiber: 10g

- Sugars: 2g

- Fat: 15g

- Saturated Fat: 2g

- Sodium: 220mg

Health Benefits:

- **Heart-Healthy Fats:** Avocado provides monounsaturated fats that support cardiovascular health.

- **High Fiber:** Whole grain bread and avocado contribute to a high fiber intake, aiding in blood sugar control and digestion.

- **Nutrient-Rich:** Avocado offers vitamins and minerals such as potassium and vitamin E, essential for overall health.

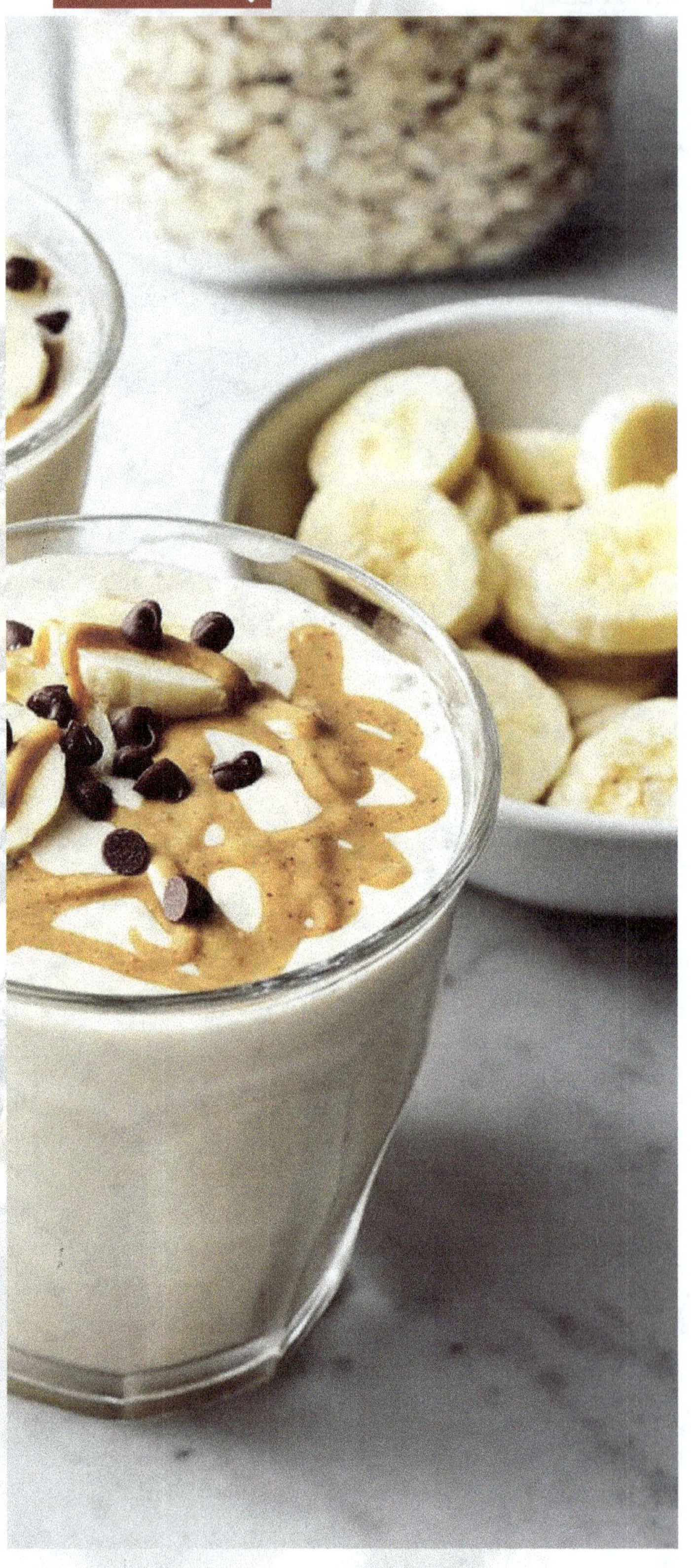

Peanut Butter Banana Smoothie

- **Preparation Time:** 5 minutes
- **Cooking Time:** None
- **Serving:** 1

Ingredients:

- 1 medium banana, preferably frozen
- 1 tablespoon natural peanut butter (no added sugar)
- 1/2 cup unsweetened almond milk
- 1/2 cup Greek yogurt (plain, non-fat)
- 1 tablespoon chia seeds
- 1/4 teaspoon cinnamon
- A few ice cubes (optional)

Procedure:

1. Peel and slice the banana if not already done.
2. In a blender, combine the banana, peanut butter, almond milk, Greek yogurt, chia seeds, and cinnamon.
3. Blend until smooth. If you prefer a thicker smoothie, add a few ice cubes and blend again until smooth.
4. Pour into a glass and enjoy immediately.

Nutritional Values (per serving):

- Calories: 300
- Protein: 15g
- Carbohydrates: 35g
- Fiber: 8g
- Sugars: 18g (natural sugars from banana)
- Fat: 12g
- Saturated Fat: 2g
- Sodium: 150mg

Health Benefits:

- **Blood Sugar Management:** The fiber from the banana and chia seeds helps slow the absorption of sugars, maintaining stable blood sugar levels.
- **Protein-Rich:** Greek yogurt and peanut butter provide a significant amount of protein, which is essential for muscle maintenance and satiety.
- **Healthy Fats:** Peanut butter and chia seeds offer healthy fats that support heart health and provide sustained energy.
- **High Fiber:** This smoothie is high in fiber, promoting good digestion and keeping you feeling full longer.

CHAPTER 3

3

LUNCHES TO SUSTAIN YOUR ENERGY

Grilled Chicken and Veggie Wrap

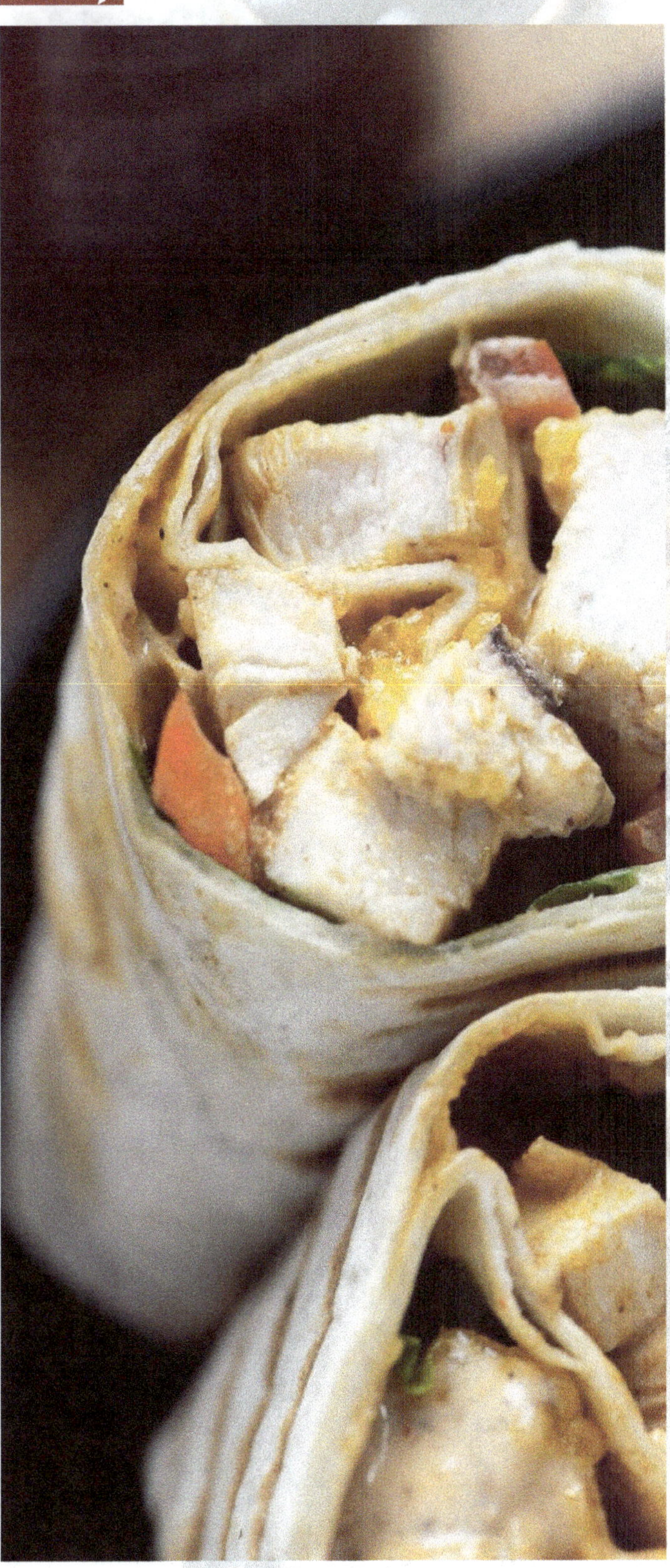

- **Preparation Time:** 10 minutes
- **Cooking Time:** 15 minutes
- **Serving:** 1

Ingredients:

- 1 whole grain tortilla
- 1 boneless, skinless chicken breast (about 4 ounces)
- 1/4 cup bell pepper, sliced (red or green)
- 1/4 cup zucchini, sliced
- 1/4 cup red onion, sliced
- 1 tablespoon olive oil
- 1/4 teaspoon black pepper
- 1/4 teaspoon salt
- 1/4 teaspoon garlic powder
- 1 tablespoon hummus
- Handful of fresh spinach leaves

Procedure:

1. Preheat the grill to medium-high heat.
2. Brush the chicken breast with olive oil and season with black pepper, salt, and garlic powder.
3. Grill the chicken for about 6-7 minutes on each side, or until fully cooked. Let it rest for a few minutes, then slice into strips.
4. While the chicken is grilling, toss the bell pepper, zucchini, and red onion in a little olive oil and grill for about 5 minutes until tender.
5. Warm the whole grain tortilla in a skillet or microwave.
6. Spread the hummus over the tortilla, then layer with spinach leaves, grilled chicken strips, and grilled vegetables.

7. Roll up the tortilla, folding in the sides to make a wrap.

8. Serve immediately and enjoy!

Nutritional Values (per serving):

- Calories: 350

- Protein: 30g

- Carbohydrates: 35g

- Fiber: 8g

- Sugars: 5g

- Fat: 12g

- Saturated Fat: 2g

- Sodium: 450mg

Health Benefits:

- **High Protein:** Grilled chicken provides lean protein essential for muscle maintenance and satiety.

- **Fiber-Rich:** Whole grain tortilla and vegetables offer high fiber content, aiding digestion and blood sugar control.

- **Healthy Fats:** Olive oil and hummus provide heart-healthy monounsaturated fats.

Quinoa and Black Bean Salad

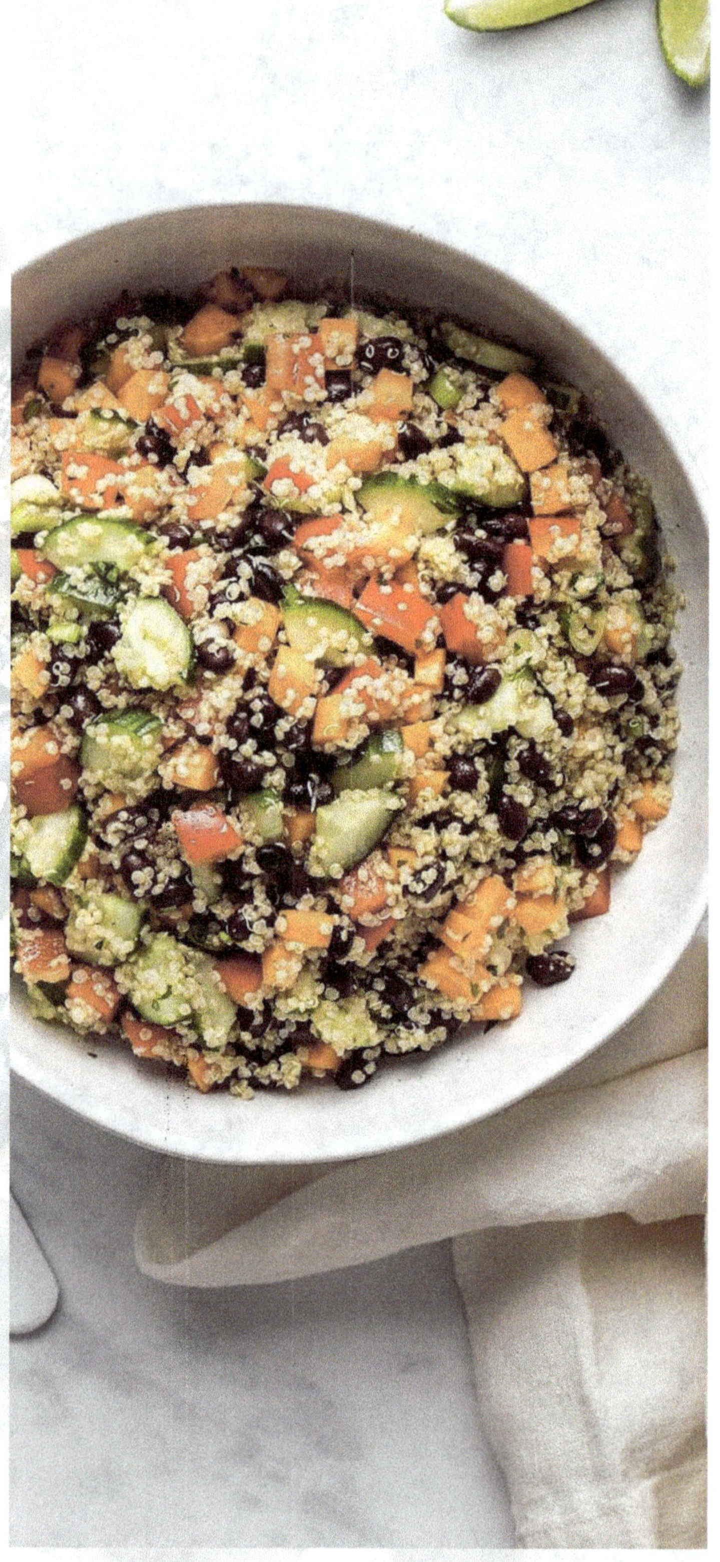

- **Preparation Time:** 15 minutes
- **Cooking Time:** 15 minutes
- **Serving:** 2

Ingredients:

- 1/2 cup quinoa
- 1 cup water
- 1 cup black beans, drained and rinsed
- 1/2 cup cherry tomatoes, halved
- 1/4 cup red onion, finely chopped
- 1/4 cup cilantro, chopped
- 1/2 avocado, diced
- 1 tablespoon olive oil
- 1 tablespoon lime juice
- 1/2 teaspoon cumin
- 1/4 teaspoon black pepper
- 1/4 teaspoon salt

Procedure:

1. Rinse quinoa under cold water.

2. In a medium saucepan, bring quinoa and water to a boil. Reduce heat, cover, and simmer for about 15 minutes, or until water is absorbed and quinoa is tender.

3. In a large bowl, combine cooked quinoa, black beans, cherry tomatoes, red onion, cilantro, and avocado.

4. In a small bowl, whisk together olive oil, lime juice, cumin, black pepper, and salt.

5. Pour the dressing over the quinoa mixture and toss to combine.

6. Serve immediately or chill in the refrigerator for a refreshing salad.

Nutritional Values (per serving):

- Calories: 320
- Protein: 10g
- Carbohydrates: 40g
- Fiber: 12g
- Sugars: 3g
- Fat: 14g
- Saturated Fat: 2g
- Sodium: 300mg

Health Benefits:

- **Blood Sugar Management:** Quinoa and black beans are low-glycemic foods that help stabilize blood sugar levels.

- **Rich in Fiber:** High fiber content from quinoa, beans, and vegetables aids digestion and promotes fullness.

- **Healthy Fats:** Avocado and olive oil provide beneficial monounsaturated fats.

Turkey and Avocado Lettuce Wraps

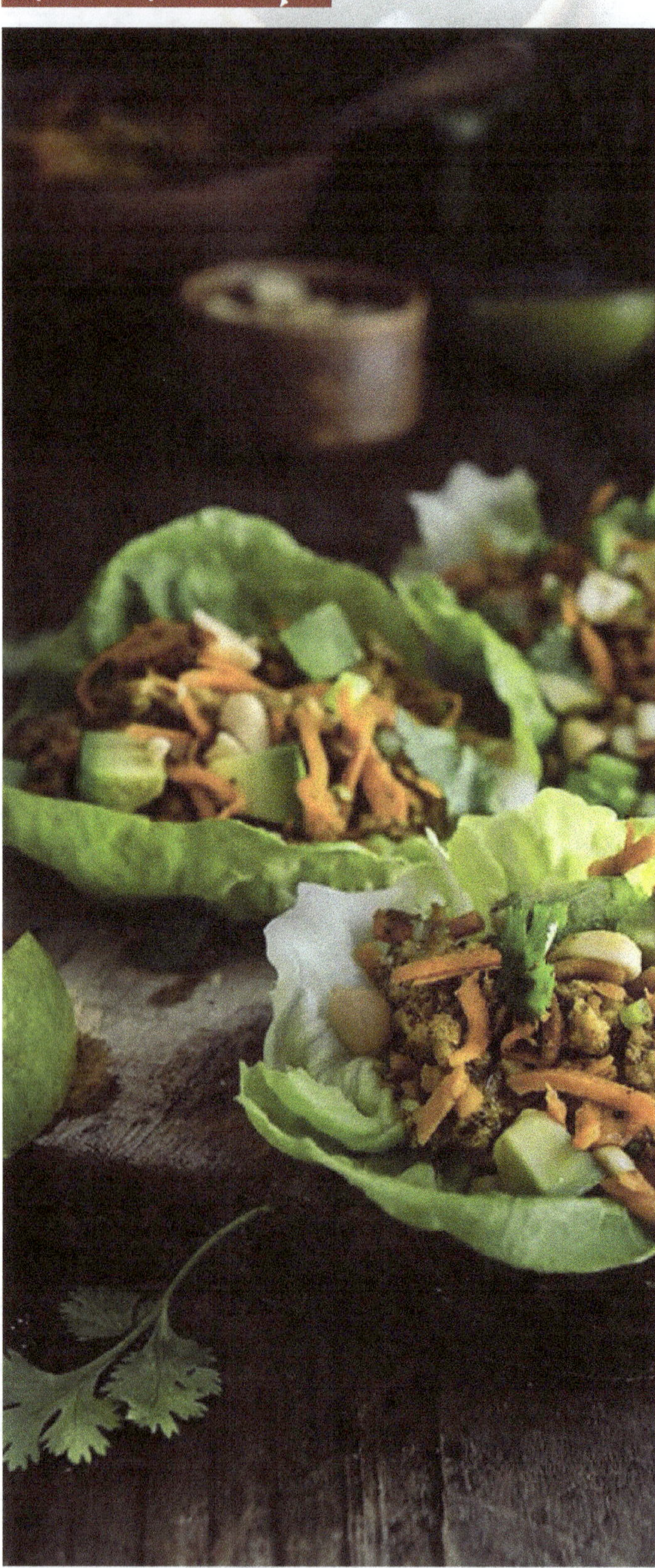

- **Preparation Time:** 10 minutes
- **Cooking Time:** 10 minutes
- **Serving:** 2

Ingredients:

- 4 large lettuce leaves (such as romaine or butter lettuce)
- 8 ounces ground turkey
- 1/2 avocado, sliced
- 1/4 cup cherry tomatoes, halved
- 1/4 cup red onion, finely chopped
- 1/4 cup cucumber, diced
- 1 tablespoon olive oil
- 1/4 teaspoon garlic powder
- 1/4 teaspoon black pepper
- 1/4 teaspoon salt
- 1 tablespoon lime juice
- 1 tablespoon cilantro, chopped

Procedure:

1. In a skillet, heat olive oil over medium heat.

2. Add ground turkey, garlic powder, black pepper, and salt. Cook, stirring occasionally, until the turkey is fully cooked, about 8-10 minutes.

3. Remove from heat and let it cool slightly.

4. Lay out the lettuce leaves and divide the cooked turkey evenly among them.

5. Top each lettuce leaf with avocado slices, cherry tomatoes, red onion, and cucumber.

6. Drizzle lime juice over the top and sprinkle with chopped cilantro.

7. Serve immediately and enjoy!

Nutritional Values (per serving):

- Calories: 250

- Protein: 22g

- Carbohydrates: 10g

- Fiber: 5g

- Sugars: 3g

- Fat: 15g

- Saturated Fat: 3g

- Sodium: 350mg

Health Benefits:

- **Low Carb:** Lettuce wraps provide a low-carb alternative to traditional wraps, helping to manage blood sugar levels.

- **High Protein:** Lean turkey is a great source of protein, essential for muscle health and satiety.

- **Healthy Fats:** Avocado and olive oil offer heart-healthy monounsaturated fats.

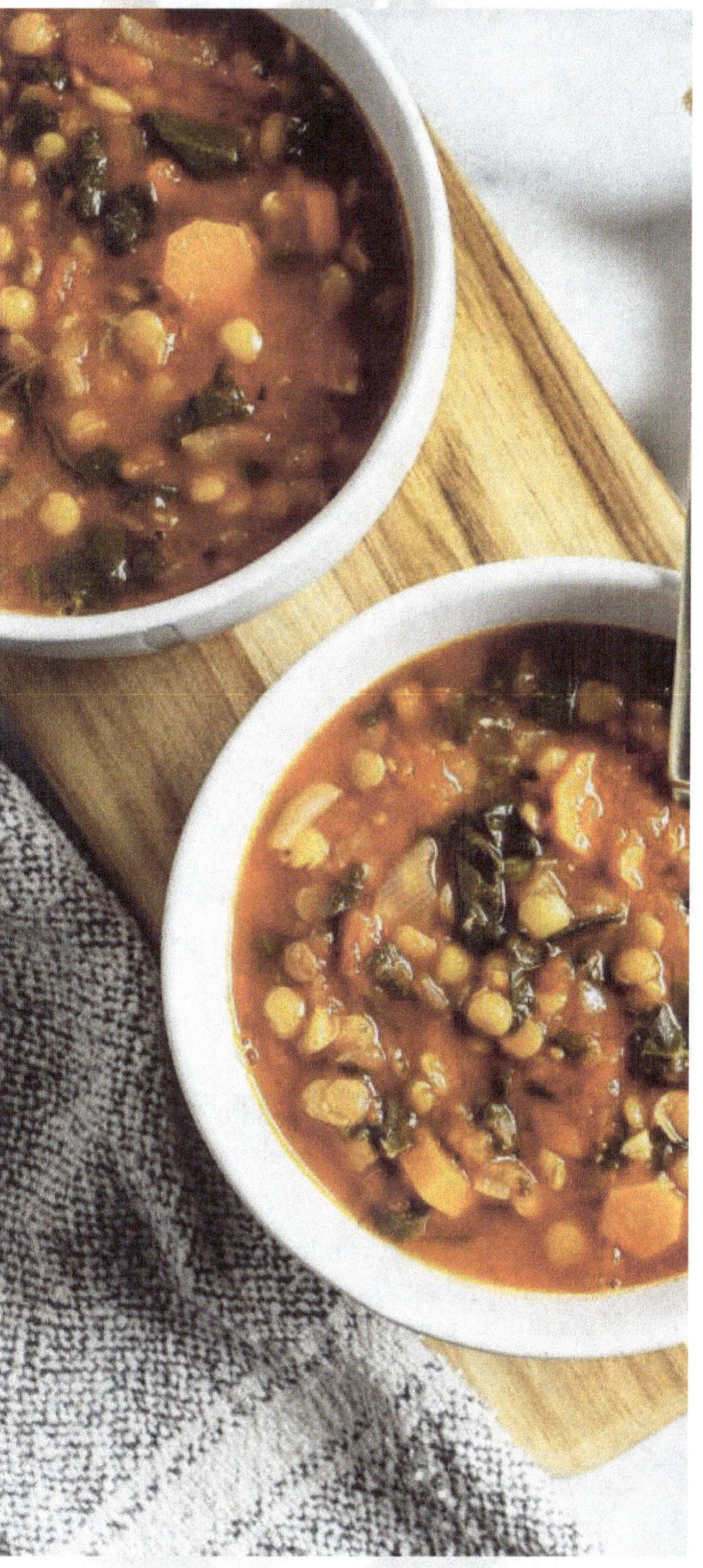

- **Preparation Time:** 10 minutes
- **Cooking Time:** 35 minutes
- **Serving:** 4

Ingredients:

- 1 cup dried lentils, rinsed
- 6 cups low-sodium vegetable broth
- 1 medium onion, diced
- 2 carrots, diced
- 2 celery stalks, diced
- 2 cloves garlic, minced
- 1 can (14.5 ounces) diced tomatoes, undrained
- 1 teaspoon cumin
- 1 teaspoon ground coriander
- 1/4 teaspoon black pepper
- 4 cups fresh spinach, chopped
- 1 tablespoon olive oil
- 1/4 teaspoon salt

Procedure:

1. In a large pot, heat olive oil over medium heat.
2. Add the onion, carrots, and celery. Sauté for about 5 minutes until the vegetables are tender.
3. Stir in the garlic, cumin, coriander, black pepper, and salt. Cook for an additional 1-2 minutes until fragrant.
4. Add the lentils, vegetable broth, and diced tomatoes. Bring to a boil.
5. Reduce heat to low, cover, and simmer for about 25 minutes, or until lentils are tender.
6. Stir in the chopped spinach and cook for an additional 5 minutes until the spinach is wilted.
7. Serve hot and enjoy!

Nutritional Values (per serving):

- Calories: 220
- Protein: 12g
- Carbohydrates: 35g
- Fiber: 15g
- Sugars: 6g
- Fat: 4g
- Saturated Fat: 0.5g
- Sodium: 320mg

Health Benefits:

- **Blood Sugar Management:** Lentils have a low glycemic index, helping to stabilize blood sugar levels.
- **High Fiber:** The soup is rich in fiber, which promotes digestive health and satiety.
- **Nutrient-Dense:** Spinach provides essential vitamins and minerals, including iron, calcium, and vitamin K.

Mediterranean Chickpea Salad

- **Preparation Time:** 15 minutes
- **Cooking Time:** None
- **Serving:** 4

Ingredients:

- 1 can (15 ounces) chickpeas, drained and rinsed
- 1 cup cherry tomatoes, halved
- 1 cucumber, diced
- 1/4 cup red onion, finely chopped
- 1/4 cup Kalamata olives, pitted and sliced
- 1/4 cup feta cheese, crumbled
- 1/4 cup fresh parsley, chopped
- 2 tablespoons olive oil
- 1 tablespoon red wine vinegar
- 1 teaspoon dried oregano
- 1/4 teaspoon black pepper
- 1/4 teaspoon salt

Procedure:

1. In a large bowl, combine chickpeas, cherry tomatoes, cucumber, red onion, olives, feta cheese, and parsley.

2. In a small bowl, whisk together olive oil, red wine vinegar, dried oregano, black pepper, and salt.

3. Pour the dressing over the chickpea mixture and toss gently to combine.

4. Serve immediately or chill in the refrigerator for an hour for flavors to meld.

5. Enjoy as a main dish or a side salad.

Nutritional Values (per serving):

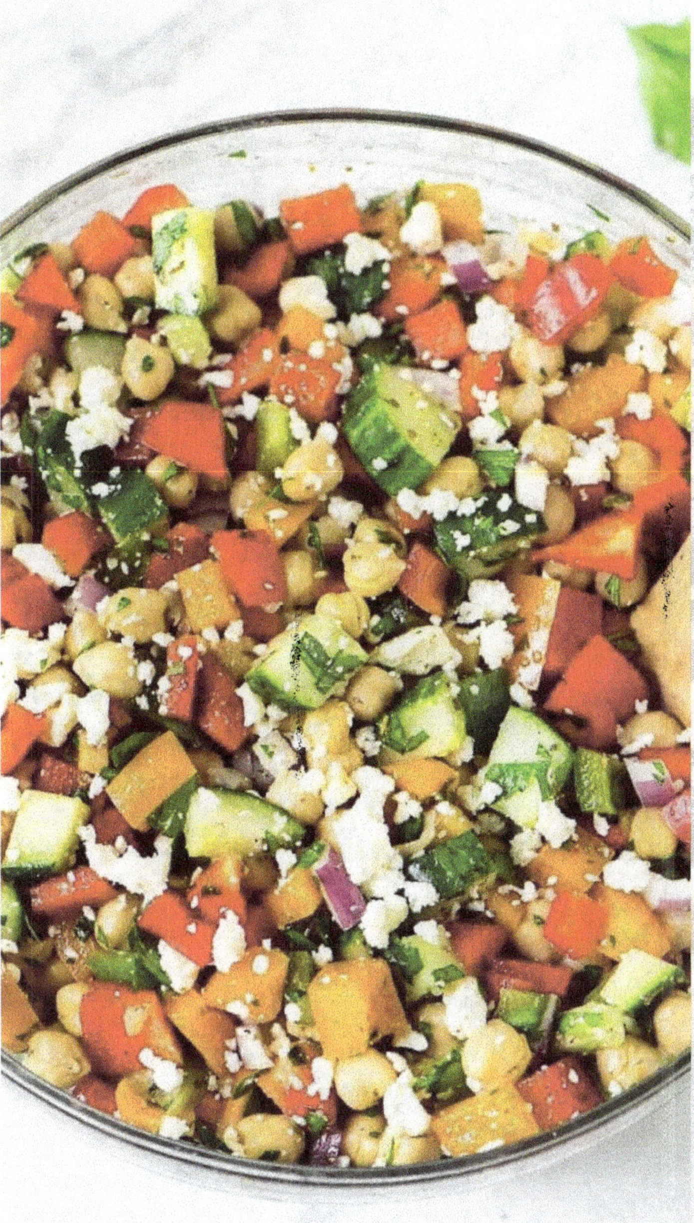

- Calories: 250

- Protein: 8g

- Carbohydrates: 24g

- Fiber: 7g

- Sugars: 4g

- Fat: 14g

- Saturated Fat: 3g

- Sodium: 400mg

Health Benefits:

- **Low Glycemic Index:** Chickpeas have a low glycemic index, helping to keep blood sugar levels stable.

- **Heart Health:** Olive oil and olives provide monounsaturated fats that support cardiovascular health.

- **Rich in Fiber:** The salad is high in fiber, promoting good digestion and prolonged fullness.

Shrimp and Asparagus Stir-Fry

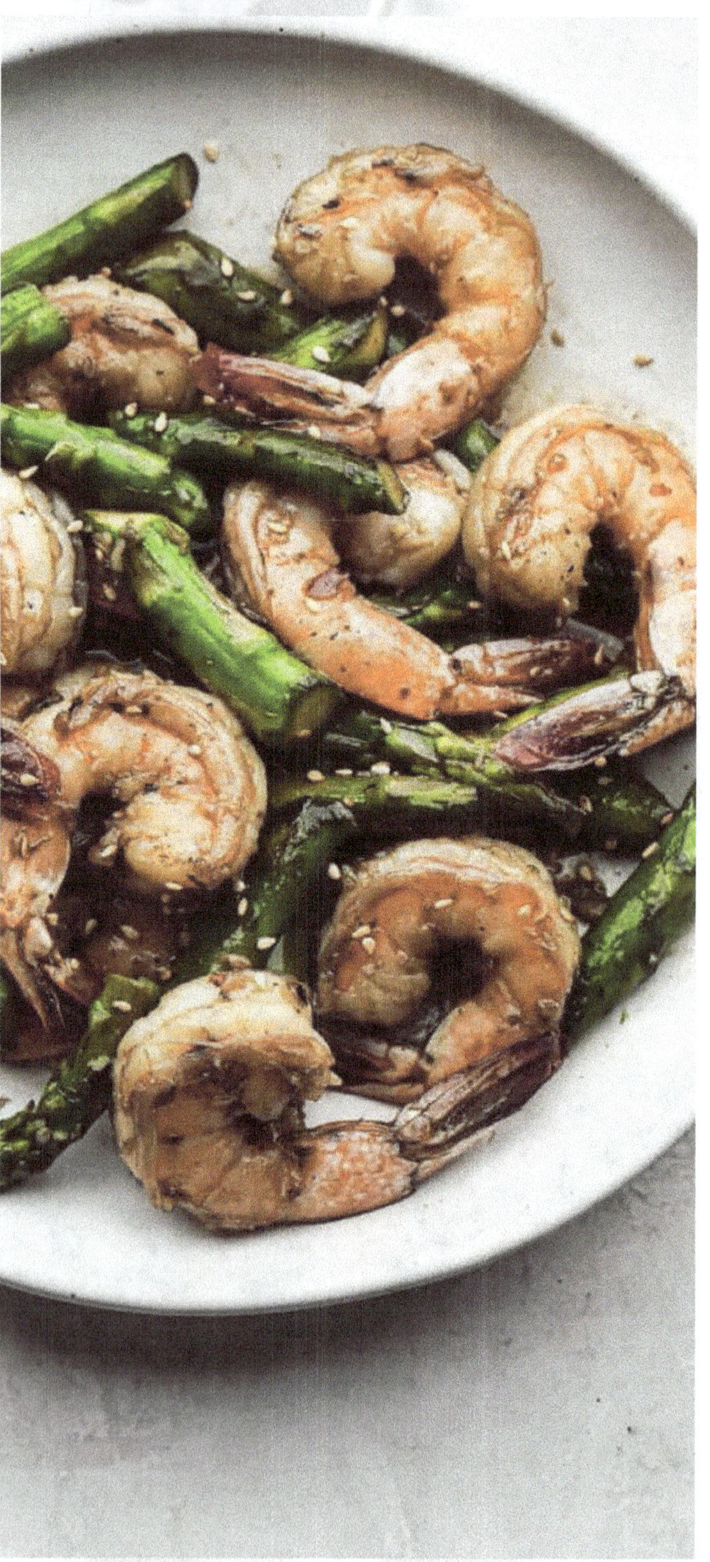

- **Preparation Time:** 10 minutes
- **Cooking Time:** 10 minutes
- **Serving:** 2

Ingredients:

- 12 ounces shrimp, peeled and deveined
- 1 bunch asparagus, trimmed and cut into 2-inch pieces
- 1 red bell pepper, sliced
- 2 cloves garlic, minced
- 1 tablespoon soy sauce (low sodium)
- 1 tablespoon olive oil
- 1 tablespoon lemon juice
- 1/4 teaspoon black pepper
- 1/4 teaspoon red pepper flakes (optional)

Procedure:

1. Heat olive oil in a large skillet or wok over medium-high heat.
2. Add garlic and cook for about 1 minute until fragrant.
3. Add shrimp to the skillet and cook for 2-3 minutes until they start to turn pink.
4. Add asparagus and red bell pepper, and stir-fry for an additional 3-4 minutes until vegetables are tender-crisp.
5. Stir in soy sauce, lemon juice, black pepper, and red pepper flakes (if using).
6. Cook for another 2 minutes until everything is well combined and heated through.
7. Serve immediately and enjoy!

Nutritional Values (per serving):

- Calories: 250
- Protein: 28g
- Carbohydrates: 10g
- Fiber: 4g
- Sugars: 4g
- Fat: 12g
- Saturated Fat: 2g
- Sodium: 400mg

Health Benefits:

- **High Protein:** Shrimp provides a lean source of protein, essential for muscle maintenance and repair.
- **Low Glycemic Index:** Asparagus and bell pepper are low-glycemic vegetables, aiding in blood sugar control.
- **Antioxidant-Rich:** Asparagus and bell pepper are rich in vitamins A and C, which support immune health and reduce inflammation.

Spinach and Ricotta Stuffed Peppers

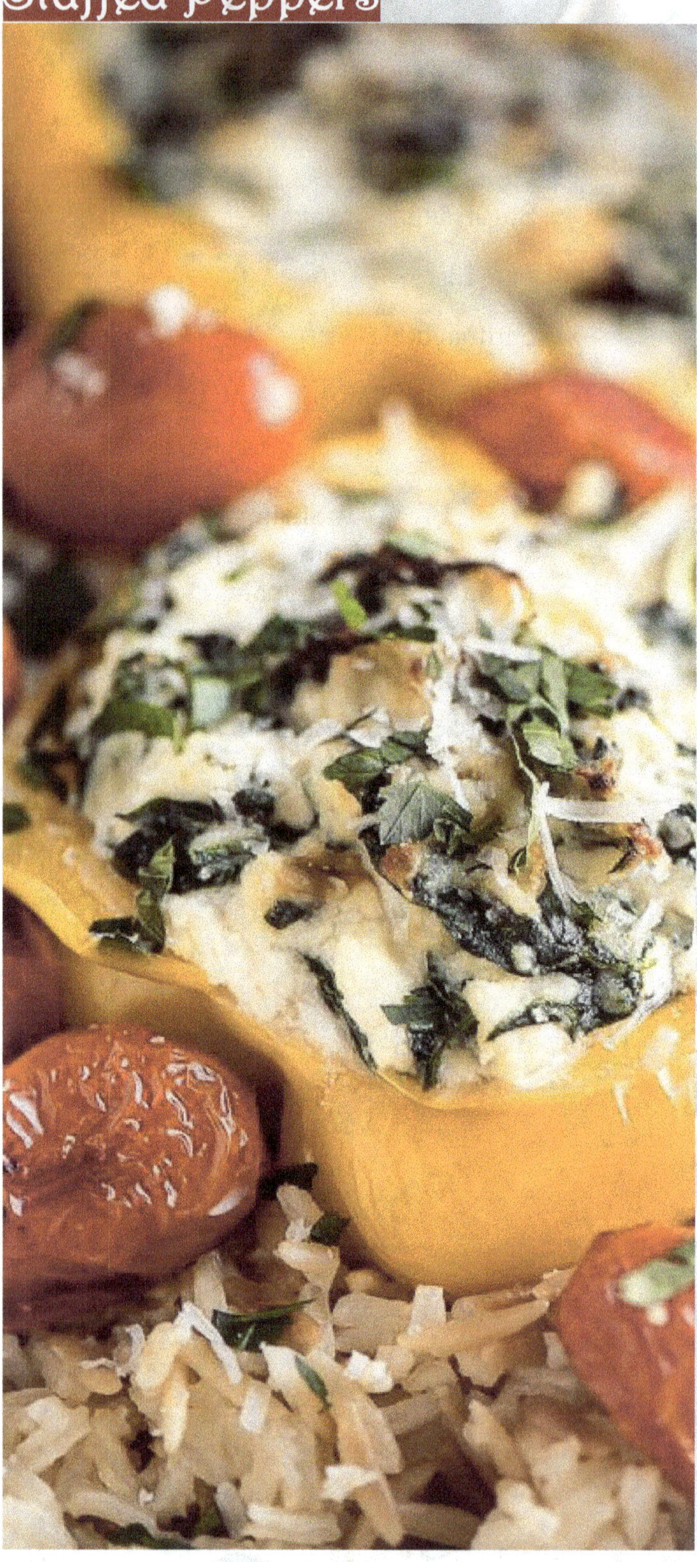

- **Preparation Time:** 15 minutes
- **Cooking Time:** 30 minutes
- **Serving:** 4

Ingredients:

- 4 large bell peppers (any color)
- 1 cup ricotta cheese (part-skim)
- 2 cups fresh spinach, chopped
- 1/4 cup grated Parmesan cheese
- 1/4 cup onion, finely chopped
- 2 cloves garlic, minced
- 1 tablespoon olive oil
- 1/4 teaspoon black pepper
- 1/4 teaspoon salt
- 1/2 teaspoon dried oregano
- 1/2 cup marinara sauce (low-sodium)

Procedure:

1. Preheat the oven to 375°F (190°C).

2. Cut the tops off the bell peppers and remove the seeds and membranes.

3. In a skillet, heat olive oil over medium heat. Add the onion and garlic and sauté until fragrant and softened, about 3-4 minutes.

4. Add the chopped spinach to the skillet and cook until wilted, about 2 minutes.

5. In a large bowl, combine the ricotta cheese, Parmesan cheese, black pepper, salt, and oregano. Stir in the sautéed spinach mixture until well combined.

6. Stuff each bell pepper with the ricotta and spinach mixture, filling them to the top.

7. Place the stuffed peppers in a baking dish and top each with a spoonful of marinara sauce.

8. Cover the dish with foil and bake for 20 minutes. Remove the foil and bake for an additional 10 minutes, until the peppers are tender and the filling is heated through.

9. Serve hot and enjoy!

Nutritional Values (per serving):

- Calories: 180
- Protein: 10g
- Carbohydrates: 12g
- Fiber: 4g
- Sugars: 6g
- Fat: 10g
- Saturated Fat: 4g
- Sodium: 320mg

Health Benefits:

- **Low Glycemic Index:** Bell peppers and spinach are low-glycemic vegetables, helping to maintain stable blood sugar levels.

- **High Fiber:** The fiber content in vegetables aids in digestion and prolongs satiety.

- **Lean Protein:** Ricotta cheese provides a source of protein, essential for muscle maintenance and repair.

Tuna and White Bean Salad

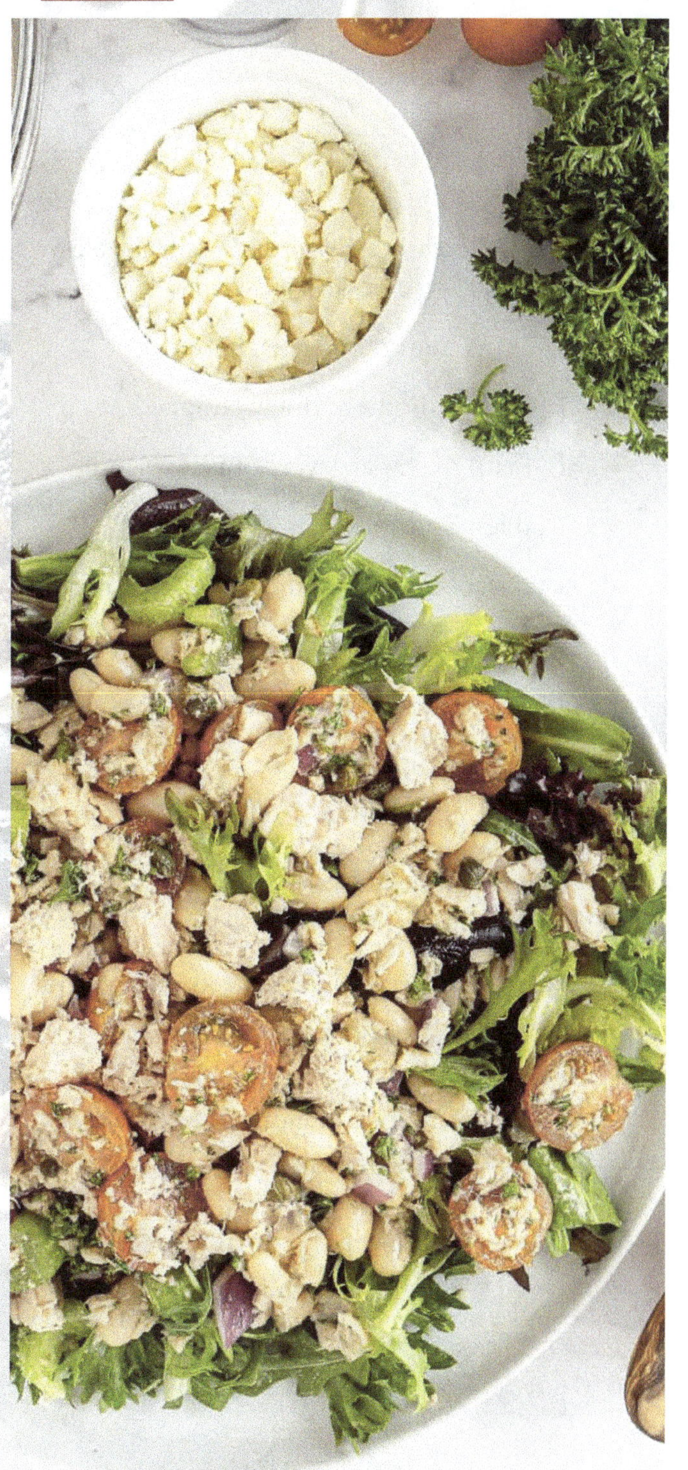

- **Preparation Time:** 10 minutes
- **Cooking Time:** None
- **Serving:** 2

Ingredients:

- 1 can (5 ounces) tuna packed in water, drained
- 1 can (15 ounces) white beans (cannellini or navy), drained and rinsed
- 1/2 cup cherry tomatoes, halved
- 1/4 cup red onion, finely chopped
- 1/4 cup fresh parsley, chopped
- 2 tablespoons olive oil
- 1 tablespoon lemon juice
- 1 teaspoon Dijon mustard
- 1/4 teaspoon black pepper
- 1/4 teaspoon salt

Procedure:

1. In a large bowl, combine the drained tuna and white beans.
2. Add the cherry tomatoes, red onion, and parsley to the bowl.
3. In a small bowl, whisk together the olive oil, lemon juice, Dijon mustard, black pepper, and salt.
4. Pour the dressing over the tuna and bean mixture, and gently toss to combine.
5. Serve immediately or chill in the refrigerator for enhanced flavors.
6. Enjoy as a main dish or a side salad.

Nutritional Values (per serving):

- Calories: 280
- Protein: 22g
- Carbohydrates: 20g
- Fiber: 8g
- Sugars: 2g
- Fat: 12g
- Saturated Fat: 2g
- Sodium: 450mg

Health Benefits:

- **High Protein:** Tuna provides a lean source of protein, essential for muscle health and satiety.
- **Rich in Fiber:** White beans add significant fiber, aiding digestion and promoting fullness.
- **Heart-Healthy Fats:** Olive oil contributes healthy monounsaturated fats, which support cardiovascular health.

CHAPTER 4

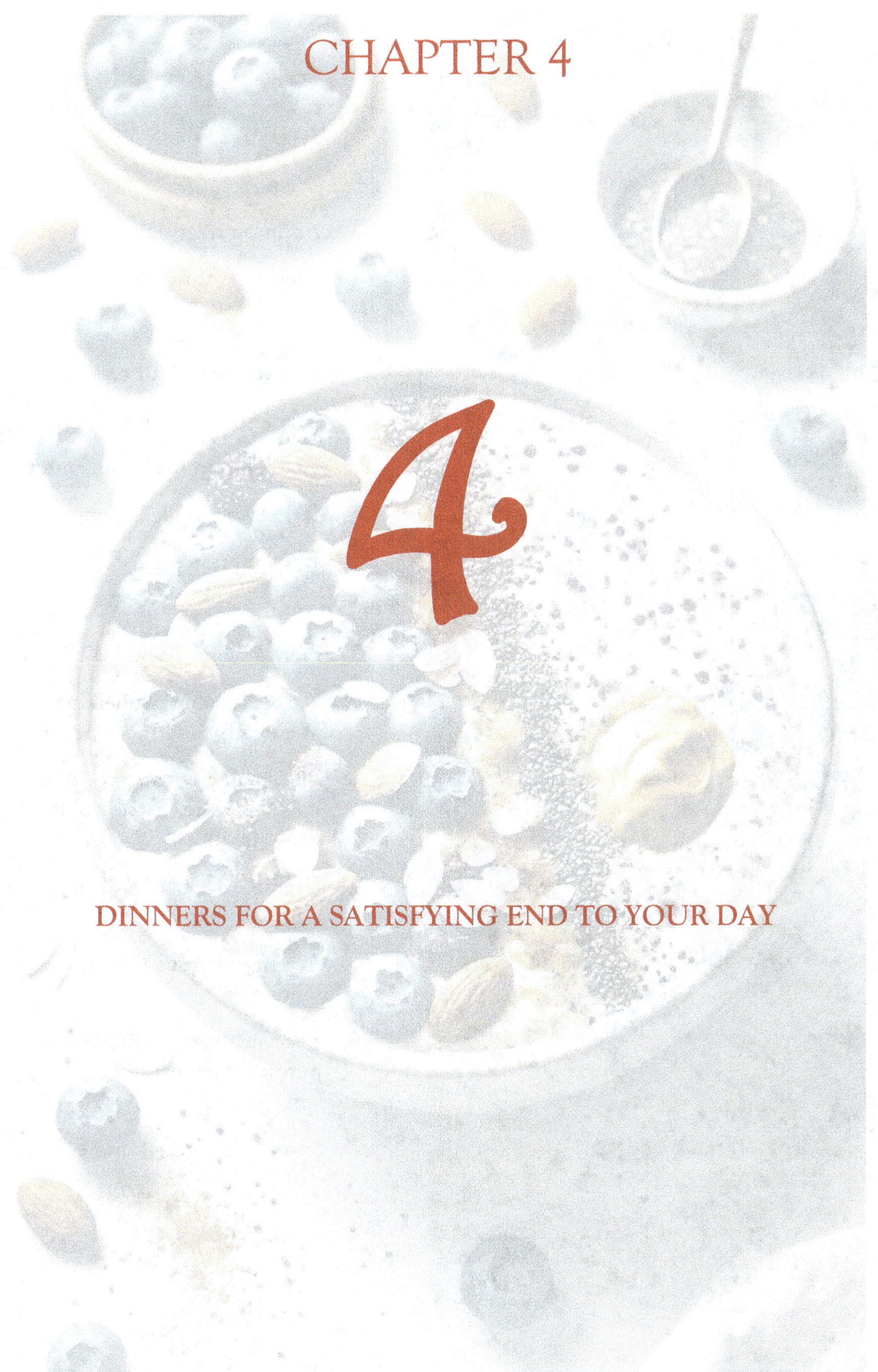

4

DINNERS FOR A SATISFYING END TO YOUR DAY

Baked Lemon Herb Salmon

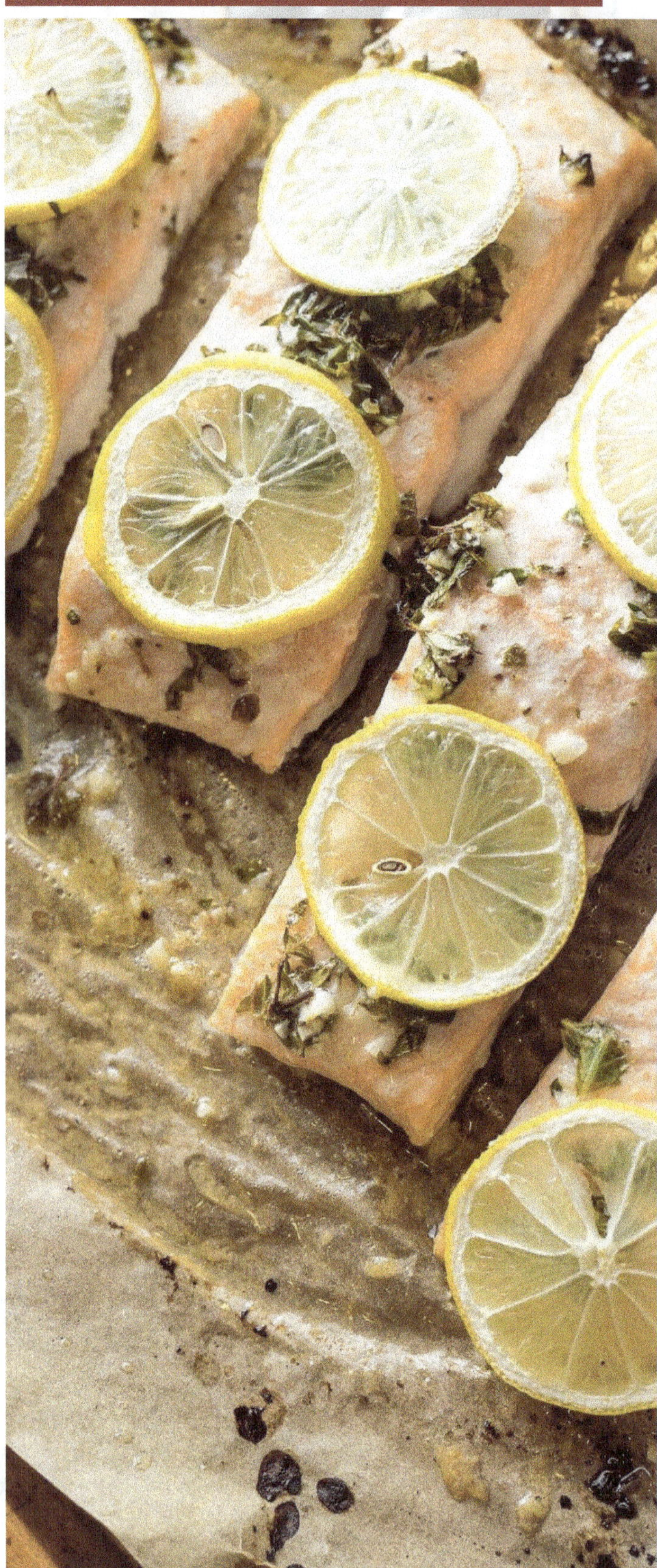

- **Preparation Time:** 10 minutes
- **Cooking Time:** 20 minutes
- **Serving:** 2

Ingredients:

- 2 salmon fillets (about 6 ounces each)
- 1 lemon, thinly sliced
- 2 tablespoons olive oil
- 2 cloves garlic, minced
- 1 tablespoon fresh parsley, chopped
- 1 tablespoon fresh dill, chopped
- 1/4 teaspoon black pepper
- 1/4 teaspoon salt

Procedure:

1. Preheat your oven to 375°F (190°C).
2. Place the salmon fillets on a baking sheet lined with parchment paper.
3. In a small bowl, mix together the olive oil, minced garlic, parsley, dill, black pepper, and salt.
4. Drizzle the olive oil mixture over the salmon fillets.
5. Arrange lemon slices on top of the salmon.
6. Bake in the preheated oven for about 20 minutes, or until the salmon flakes easily with a fork.
7. Serve immediately and enjoy!

Nutritional Values (per serving):

- Calories: 350
- Protein: 28g
- Carbohydrates: 2g

- Fiber: 1g

- Sugars: 0g

- Fat: 25g

- Saturated Fat: 4g

- Sodium: 300mg

Health Benefits:

- **Rich in Omega-3:** Salmon is high in omega-3 fatty acids, which help reduce inflammation and improve heart health.

- **High Protein:** Provides lean protein, essential for muscle maintenance and repair.

- **Low Glycemic Index:** Supports stable blood sugar levels.

Chicken and Broccoli Stir-Fry

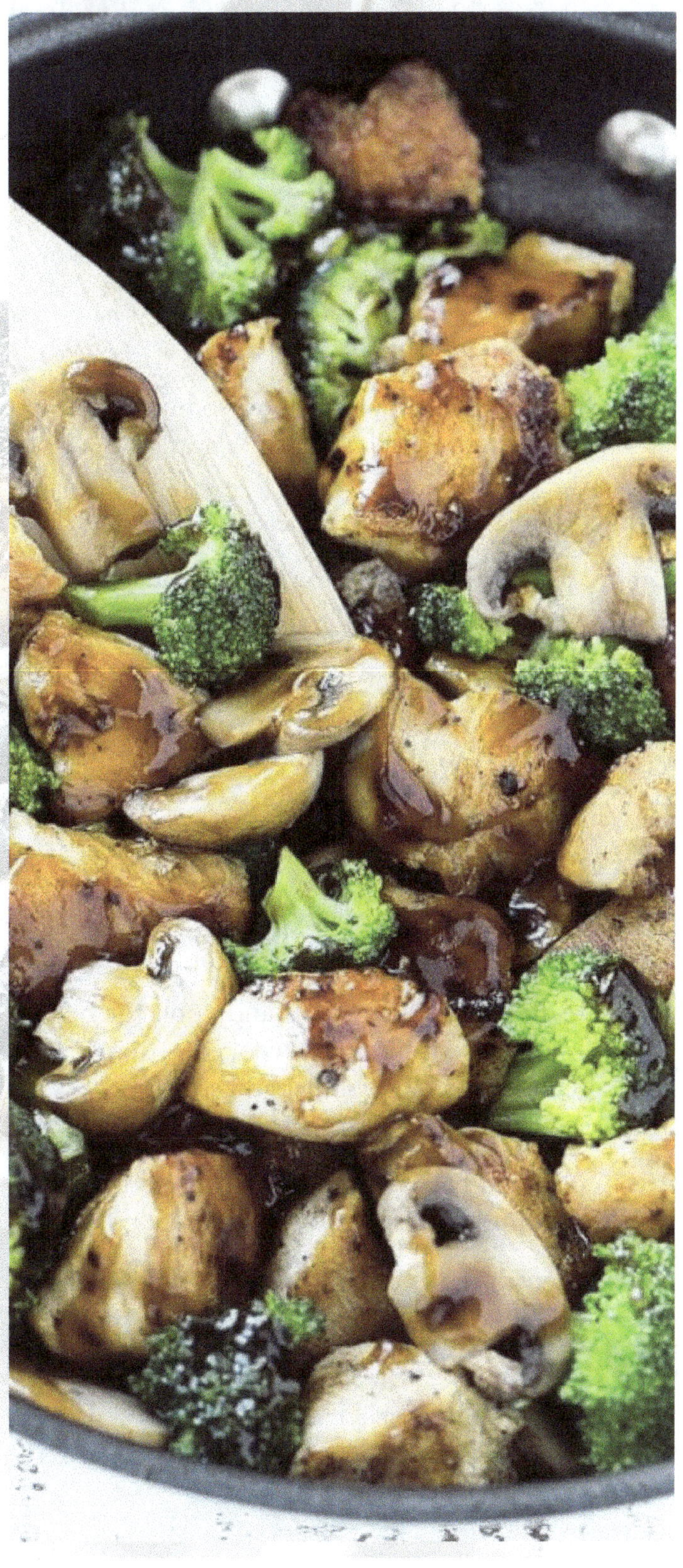

- **Preparation Time:** 10 minutes
- **Cooking Time:** 15 minutes
- **Serving:** 2

Ingredients:

- 2 boneless, skinless chicken breasts (about 6 ounces each), sliced into thin strips
- 2 cups broccoli florets
- 1 red bell pepper, sliced
- 2 cloves garlic, minced
- 1 tablespoon soy sauce (low sodium)
- 1 tablespoon olive oil
- 1 tablespoon oyster sauce
- 1 tablespoon water
- 1 teaspoon cornstarch
- 1/4 teaspoon black pepper

Procedure:

1. In a small bowl, mix the water and cornstarch to create a slurry. Set aside.
2. Heat olive oil in a large skillet or wok over medium-high heat.
3. Add the chicken strips and cook for 5-7 minutes until fully cooked. Remove chicken from the skillet and set aside.
4. In the same skillet, add the garlic, broccoli, and red bell pepper. Stir-fry for about 3-4 minutes until vegetables are tender-crisp.
5. Return the chicken to the skillet. Add the soy sauce, oyster sauce, and black pepper. Stir to combine.
6. Pour the cornstarch slurry into the skillet and cook for another 2-3 minutes until the sauce thickens.
7. Serve immediately and enjoy!

Nutritional Values (per serving):

- Calories: 300
- Protein: 32g
- Carbohydrates: 12g
- Fiber: 4g
- Sugars: 5g
- Fat: 14g
- Saturated Fat: 2g
- Sodium: 400mg

Health Benefits:

- **High Protein:** Chicken provides lean protein, essential for muscle health.
- **Rich in Fiber:** Broccoli and bell pepper add fiber, aiding digestion and promoting fullness.
- **Low Glycemic Index:** Supports stable blood sugar levels.

Beef and Vegetable Skillet

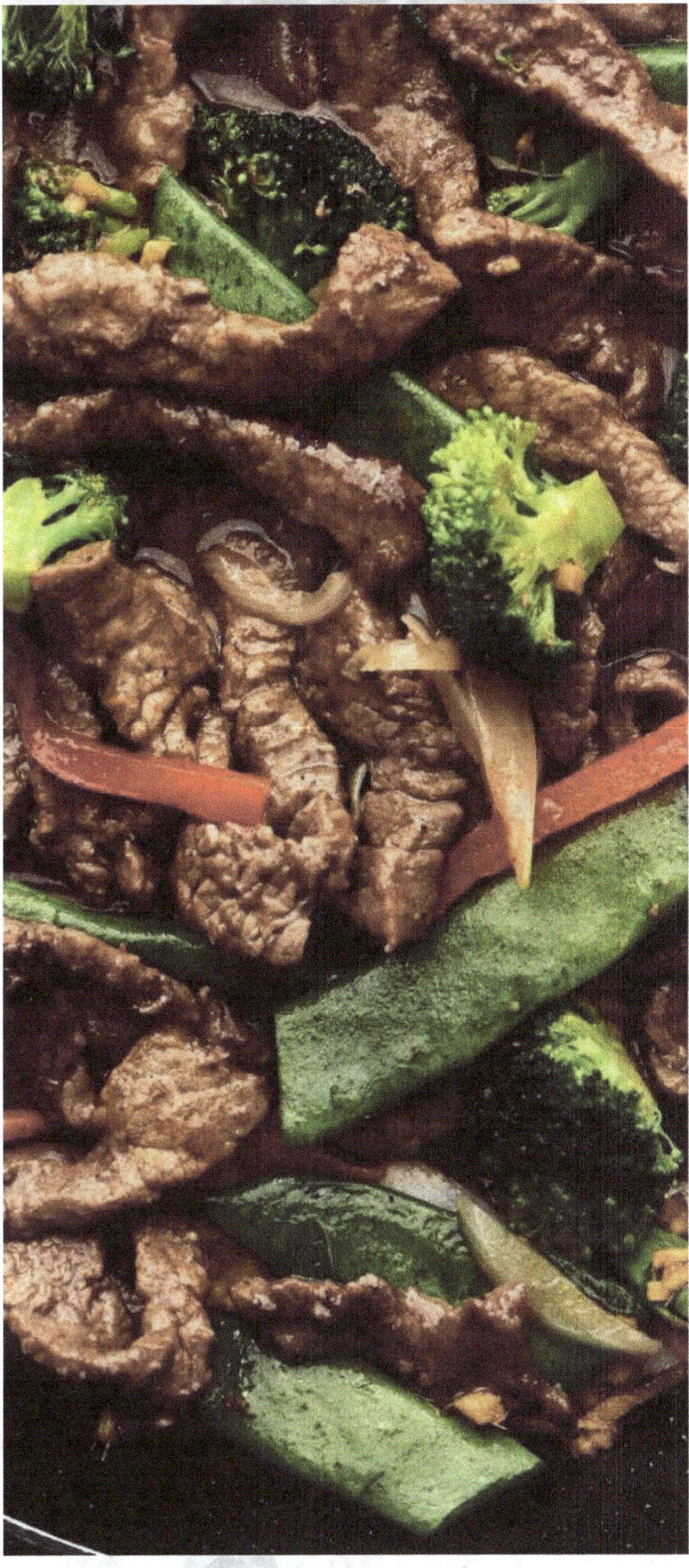

- **Preparation Time:** 10 minutes
- **Cooking Time:** 20 minutes
- **Serving:** 2

Ingredients:

- 8 ounces lean beef sirloin, thinly sliced
- 1 cup zucchini, sliced
- 1 cup mushrooms, sliced
- 1/2 cup red onion, sliced
- 1 cup cherry tomatoes, halved
- 2 cloves garlic, minced
- 2 tablespoons olive oil
- 1 tablespoon balsamic vinegar
- 1/4 teaspoon black pepper
- 1/4 teaspoon salt
- 1 teaspoon dried thyme

Procedure:

1. Heat 1 tablespoon of olive oil in a large skillet over medium-high heat.

2. Add the sliced beef and cook for about 5-7 minutes until browned and cooked through. Remove beef from the skillet and set aside.

3. In the same skillet, add the remaining tablespoon of olive oil, garlic, zucchini, mushrooms, red onion, and cherry tomatoes. Cook for about 5-7 minutes until vegetables are tender.

4. Return the beef to the skillet and add the balsamic vinegar, black pepper, salt, and dried thyme. Stir to combine and cook for another 2-3 minutes until everything is heated through.

5. Serve immediately and enjoy!

Nutritional Values (per serving):

- Calories: 350
- Protein: 28g
- Carbohydrates: 14g
- Fiber: 5g
- Sugars: 6g
- Fat: 18g
- Saturated Fat: 4g
- Sodium: 400mg

Health Benefits:

- **High Protein:** Lean beef provides a good source of protein, vital for muscle maintenance.
- **Rich in Fiber:** Vegetables contribute to high fiber content, aiding digestion and satiety.
- **Low Glycemic Index:** Helps maintain stable blood sugar levels.

Stuffed Zucchini Boats

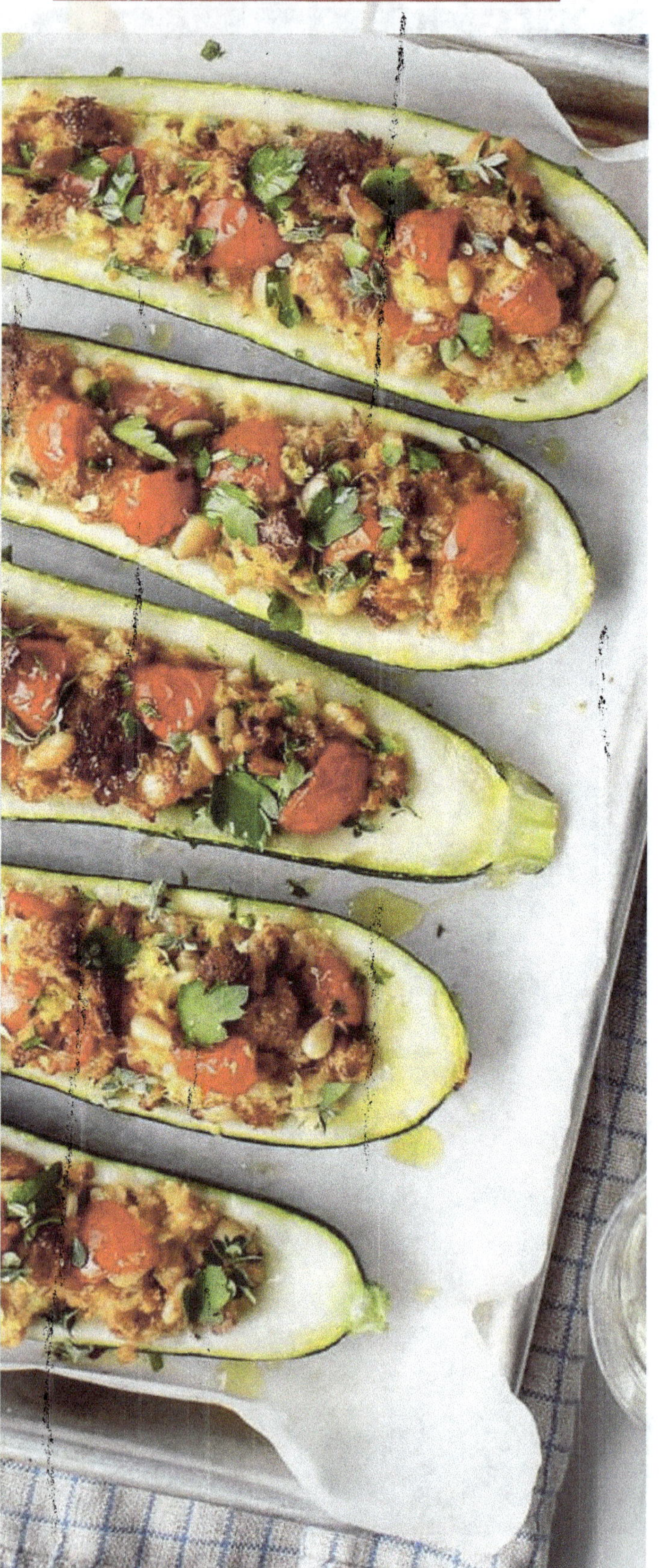

- **Preparation Time:** 15 minutes
- **Cooking Time:** 25 minutes
- **Serving:** 4

Ingredients:

- 4 medium zucchinis
- 1/2 pound lean ground turkey
- 1/2 cup onion, finely chopped
- 1/2 cup bell pepper, finely chopped
- 1 cup diced tomatoes (canned or fresh)
- 2 cloves garlic, minced
- 1/2 cup shredded mozzarella cheese (part-skim)
- 1 tablespoon olive oil
- 1 teaspoon Italian seasoning
- 1/4 teaspoon black pepper
- 1/4 teaspoon salt

Procedure:

1. Preheat your oven to 375°F (190°C).
2. Slice the zucchinis in half lengthwise and scoop out the flesh to create boats, leaving a 1/4-inch thick shell. Chop the scooped-out zucchini flesh and set aside.
3. In a large skillet, heat olive oil over medium heat. Add the onion, bell pepper, and garlic, and sauté until softened, about 3-4 minutes.
4. Add the ground turkey and cook until browned, breaking it up with a spoon, about 5-7 minutes.
5. Stir in the chopped zucchini flesh, diced tomatoes, Italian seasoning, black pepper, and salt. Cook for an additional 5 minutes until the mixture is well combined and heated through.
6. Place the zucchini boats in a baking dish and fill each with the turkey mixture.
7. Top with shredded mozzarella cheese.
8. Bake in the preheated oven for 20-25 minutes, until the zucchini is tender and the cheese is melted and golden.
9. Serve hot and enjoy!

Nutritional Values (per serving):

- Calories: 220
- Protein: 20g
- Carbohydrates: 10g
- Fiber: 3g
- Sugars: 5g
- Fat: 12g
- Saturated Fat: 3g
- Sodium: 380mg

Health Benefits:

- **Low Glycemic Index:** Zucchini and lean turkey help maintain stable blood sugar levels.
- **High Protein:** Provides essential protein for muscle maintenance and satiety.
- **Rich in Fiber:** Vegetables add fiber, aiding digestion and promoting fullness.

Turkey Meatballs with Zucchini Noodles

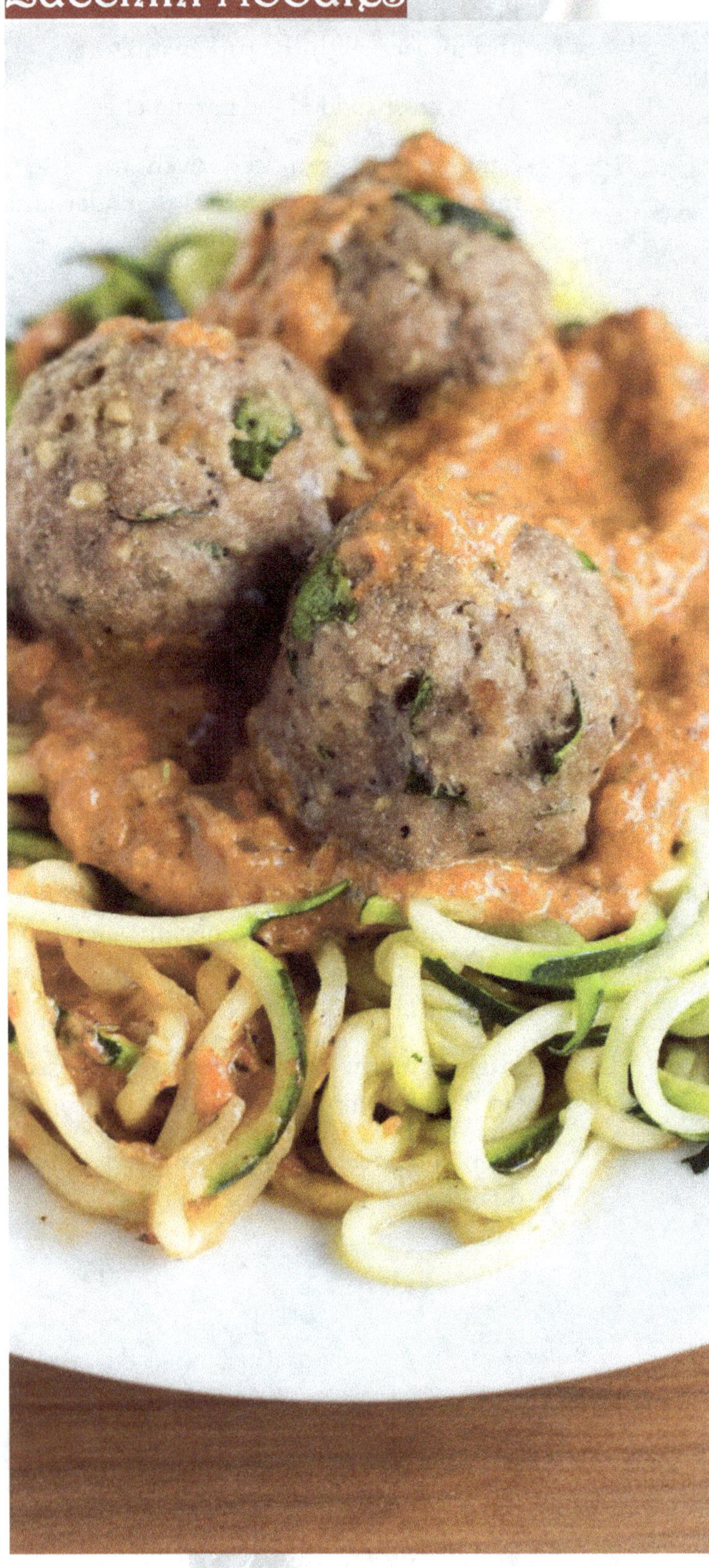

- **Preparation Time:** 15 minutes
- **Cooking Time:** 20 minutes
- **Serving:** 4

Ingredients:

- 1 pound lean ground turkey

- 1/4 cup grated Parmesan cheese

- 1/4 cup whole wheat breadcrumbs

- 1 large egg, beaten

- 2 cloves garlic, minced

- 1 tablespoon fresh parsley, chopped

- 1/4 teaspoon black pepper

- 1/4 teaspoon salt

- 4 medium zucchinis, spiralized into noodles

- 1 tablespoon olive oil

- 1 cup marinara sauce (low-sodium)

Procedure:

1. Preheat your oven to 400°F (200°C).

2. In a large bowl, combine ground turkey, Parmesan cheese, breadcrumbs, egg, garlic, parsley, black pepper, and salt. Mix well.

3. Form the mixture into small meatballs, about 1 inch in diameter, and place them on a baking sheet lined with parchment paper.

4. Bake the meatballs in the preheated oven for 15-20 minutes, until fully cooked and golden brown.

5. While the meatballs are baking, heat olive oil in a large skillet over medium heat. Add the zucchini noodles and sauté for about 3-4 minutes until tender.

6. Warm the marinara sauce in a small saucepan over low heat.

7. Serve the turkey meatballs over the zucchini noodles, topped with marinara sauce.

8. Enjoy!

Nutritional Values (per serving):

- Calories: 300

- Protein: 28g

- Carbohydrates: 14g

- Fiber: 5g

- Sugars: 7g

- Fat: 14g

- Saturated Fat: 3g

- Sodium: 450mg

Health Benefits:

- **High Protein:** Lean turkey provides essential protein for muscle health.

- **Low Glycemic Index:** Zucchini noodles help maintain stable blood sugar levels.

- **Rich in Fiber:** Zucchini and marinara sauce add fiber, promoting good digestion and satiety.

Grilled Pork Chops with Apple Slaw

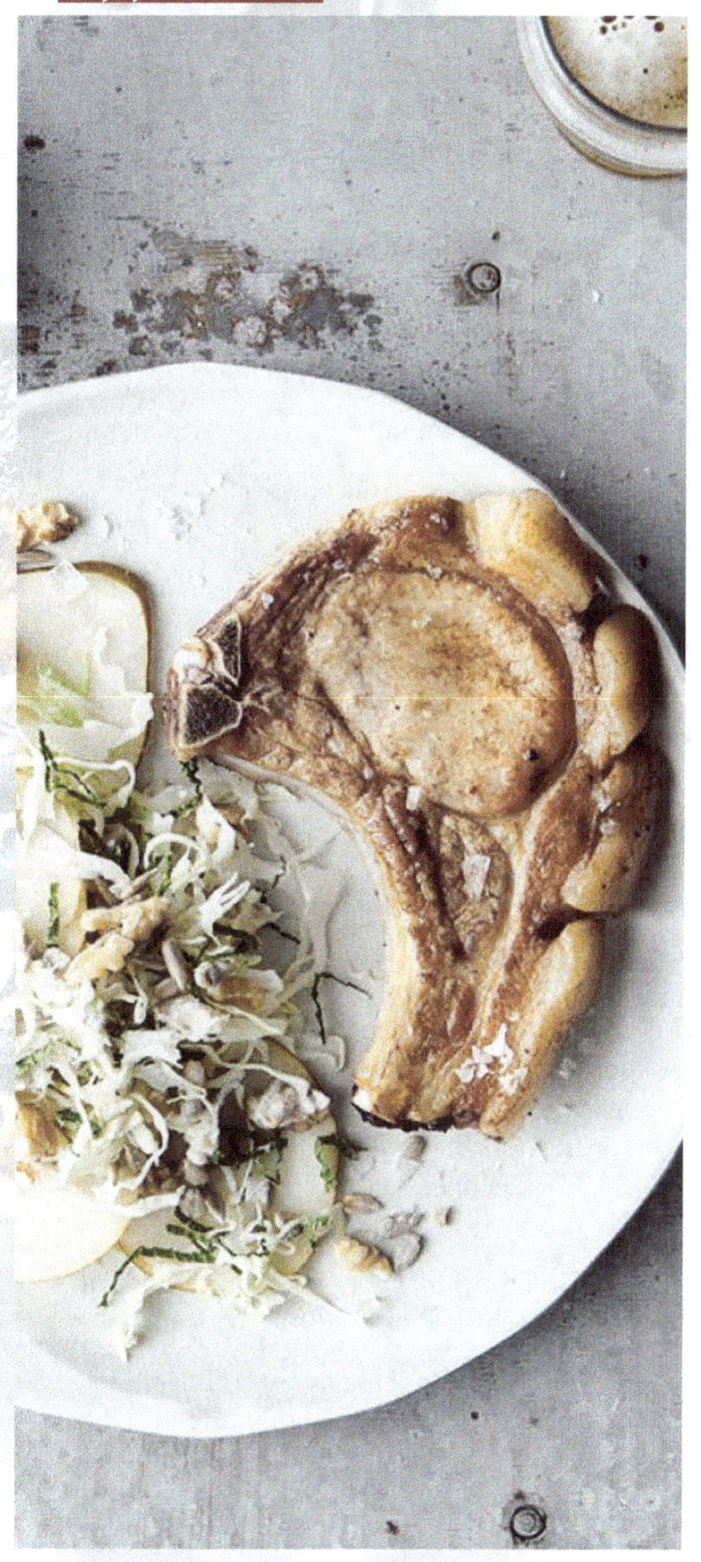

- **Preparation Time:** 15 minutes
- **Cooking Time:** 15 minutes
- **Serving:** 2

Ingredients:

- 2 bone-in pork chops (about 6 ounces each)
- 1 tablespoon olive oil
- 1 teaspoon paprika
- 1/2 teaspoon black pepper
- 1/2 teaspoon salt
- 1/4 teaspoon garlic powder
- 2 cups shredded cabbage
- 1 apple, thinly sliced
- 1/4 cup red onion, thinly sliced
- 2 tablespoons apple cider vinegar
- 1 tablespoon Dijon mustard
- 1 tablespoon honey or stevia
- 1/4 teaspoon black pepper
- 1/4 teaspoon salt

Procedure:

1. Preheat your grill to medium-high heat.
2. In a small bowl, mix olive oil, paprika, black pepper, salt, and garlic powder. Rub this mixture onto the pork chops.
3. Grill the pork chops for about 5-7 minutes on each side, or until fully cooked.
4. While the pork chops are grilling, prepare the apple slaw by combining shredded cabbage, apple slices, and red onion in a large bowl.
5. In a small bowl, whisk together apple cider vinegar, Dijon mustard, honey (or stevia), black pepper, and salt.
6. Pour the dressing over the cabbage mixture and toss to combine.
7. Serve the grilled pork chops with a generous portion of apple slaw.
8. Enjoy!

Nutritional Values (per serving):

- Calories: 400
- Protein: 30g
- Carbohydrates: 20g
- Fiber: 5g
- Sugars: 10g
- Fat: 22g
- Saturated Fat: 6g
- Sodium: 600mg

Health Benefits:

- **High Protein:** Pork chops provide essential protein for muscle health.
- **Low Glycemic Index:** Apple and cabbage are low-glycemic foods, helping to stabilize blood sugar levels.
- **Rich in Fiber:** The apple slaw adds fiber, promoting good digestion and satiety.

Vegetable and Tofu Stir-Fry

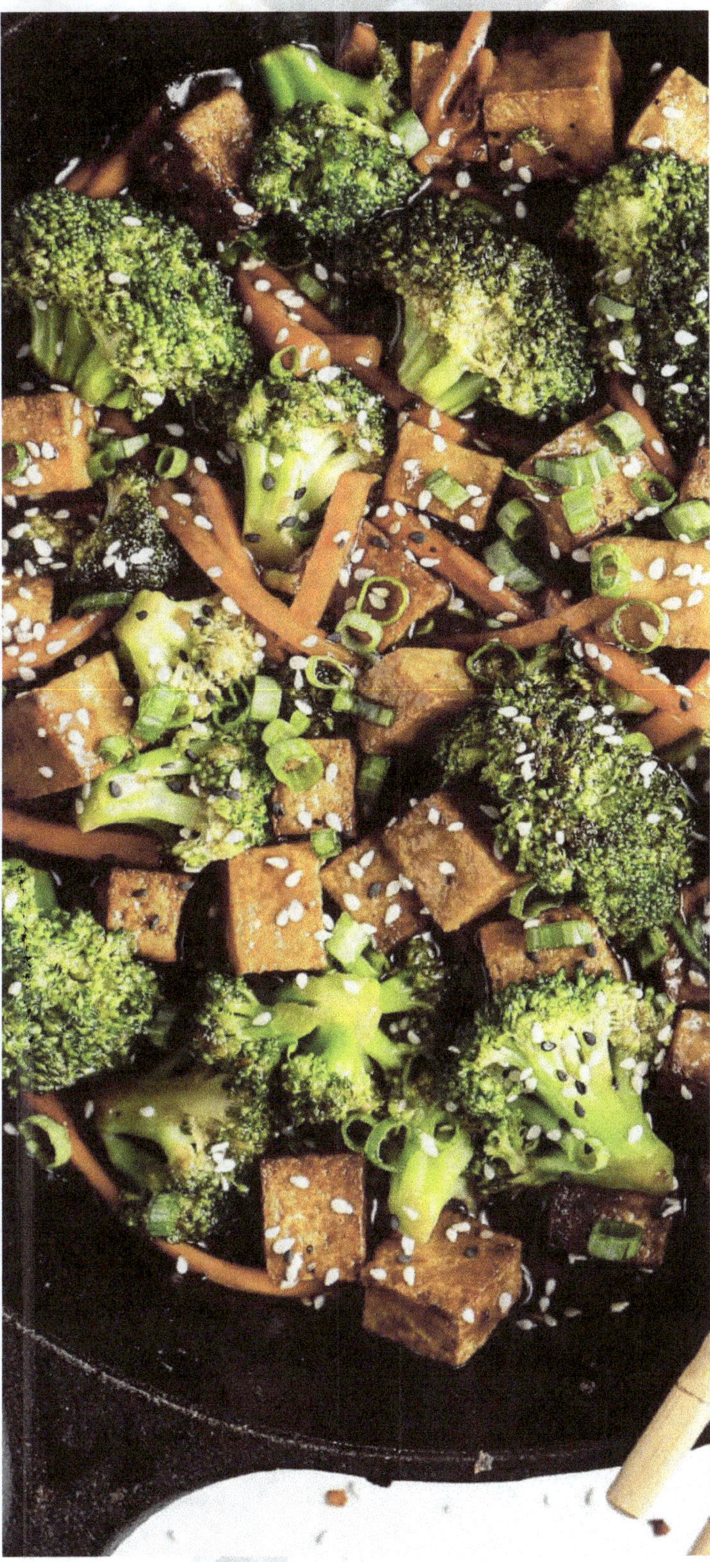

- **Preparation Time:** 15 minutes
- **Cooking Time:** 15 minutes
- **Serving:** 2

Ingredients:

- 8 ounces firm tofu, drained and cubed
- 1 cup broccoli florets
- 1 cup bell pepper, sliced
- 1 cup snap peas
- 1/2 cup carrots, thinly sliced
- 2 cloves garlic, minced
- 1 tablespoon fresh ginger, grated
- 2 tablespoons low-sodium soy sauce
- 1 tablespoon sesame oil
- 1 tablespoon olive oil
- 1 tablespoon rice vinegar
- 1 tablespoon sesame seeds
- 1/4 teaspoon black pepper
- 1/4 teaspoon salt
- 2 green onions, chopped (for garnish)

Procedure:

1. Heat olive oil in a large skillet or wok over medium-high heat.
2. Add the cubed tofu and cook for about 5 minutes, turning occasionally, until golden brown. Remove the tofu from the skillet and set aside.
3. In the same skillet, add sesame oil and heat over medium-high heat.
4. Add garlic and ginger, and sauté for 1 minute until fragrant.

5. Add broccoli, bell pepper, snap peas, and carrots. Stir-fry for about 5-7 minutes until the vegetables are tender-crisp.

6. Return the tofu to the skillet. Add soy sauce, rice vinegar, black pepper, and salt. Stir well to combine.

7. Cook for another 2 minutes until everything is heated through.

8. Sprinkle sesame seeds over the top and garnish with chopped green onions.

9. Serve immediately and enjoy!

Nutritional Values (per serving):

- Calories: 250
- Protein: 12g
- Carbohydrates: 20g
- Fiber: 6g
- Sugars: 6g
- Fat: 14g
- Saturated Fat: 2g
- Sodium: 450mg

Health Benefits:

- **High Protein:** Tofu provides plant-based protein, essential for muscle maintenance.

- **Low Glycemic Index:** Vegetables and tofu help maintain stable blood sugar levels.

- **Rich in Fiber:** Vegetables contribute to high fiber content, aiding digestion and promoting satiety.

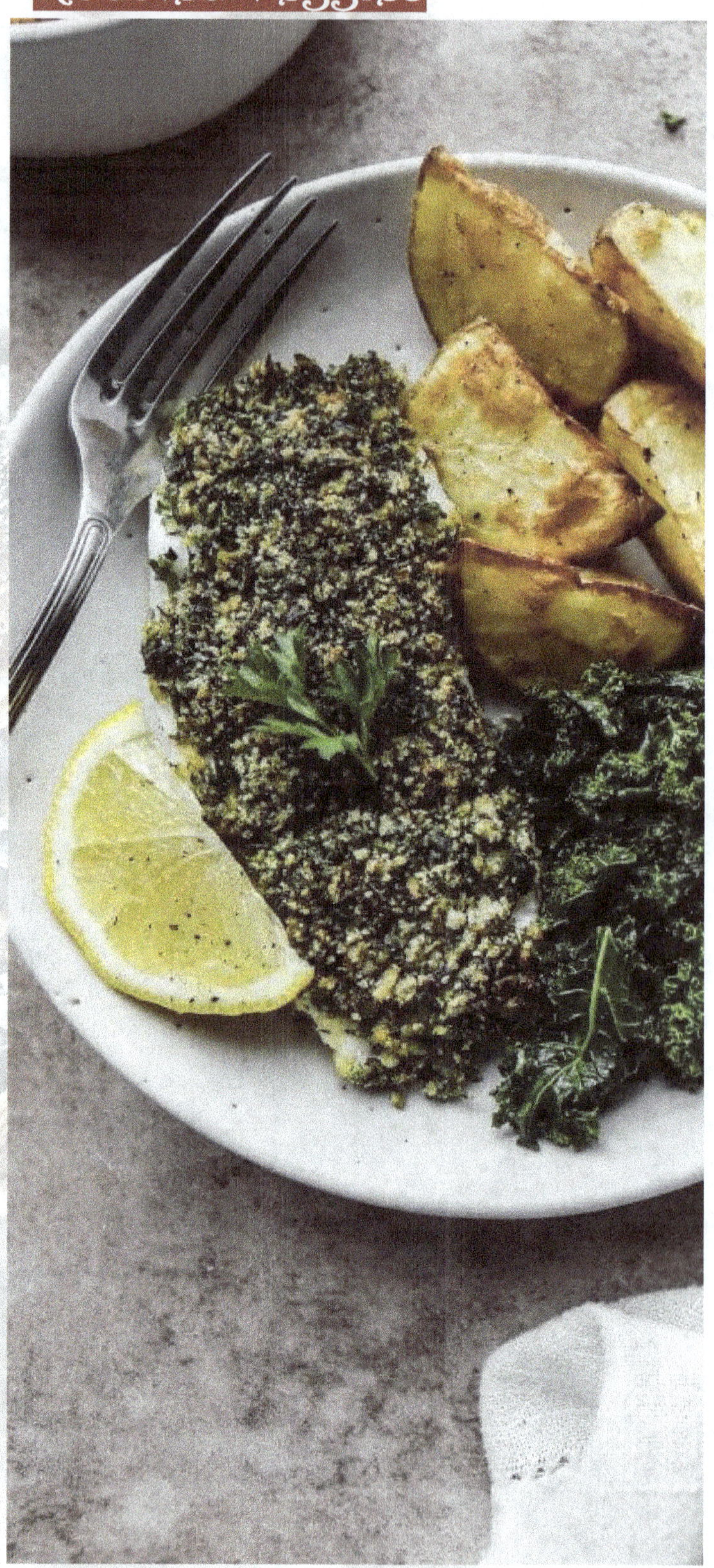

- **Preparation Time:** 15 minutes
- **Cooking Time:** 25 minutes
- **Serving:** 2

Ingredients:

- 2 cod fillets (about 6 ounces each)
- 1 tablespoon olive oil
- 1 tablespoon lemon juice
- 1 tablespoon fresh parsley, chopped
- 1 tablespoon fresh dill, chopped
- 1 teaspoon garlic powder
- 1/2 teaspoon black pepper
- 1/2 teaspoon salt
- 1 cup cherry tomatoes, halved
- 1 cup zucchini, sliced
- 1 cup red bell pepper, sliced
- 1 cup baby carrots
- 1 tablespoon balsamic vinegar

Procedure:

1. Preheat the oven to 400°F (200°C).

2. In a small bowl, mix olive oil, lemon juice, parsley, dill, garlic powder, black pepper, and salt.

3. Place the cod fillets on a baking sheet lined with parchment paper. Brush the herb mixture over the cod fillets.

4. In a separate bowl, toss cherry tomatoes, zucchini, red bell pepper, and baby carrots with balsamic vinegar and a pinch of salt and pepper.

5. Spread the vegetables around the cod fillets on the baking sheet.

6. Bake in the preheated oven for 20-25 minutes, until the cod is cooked through and flakes easily with a fork, and the vegetables are tender.

7. Serve immediately and enjoy!

Nutritional Values (per serving):

- Calories: 300
- Protein: 25g
- Carbohydrates: 18g
- Fiber: 6g
- Sugars: 10g
- Fat: 12g
- Saturated Fat: 2g
- Sodium: 450mg

Health Benefits:

- **High Protein:** Cod provides lean protein, essential for muscle maintenance and repair.

- **Low Glycemic Index:** Cod and vegetables help maintain stable blood sugar levels.

- **Rich in Fiber:** The variety of vegetables adds fiber, promoting good digestion and satiety.

CHAPTER 5

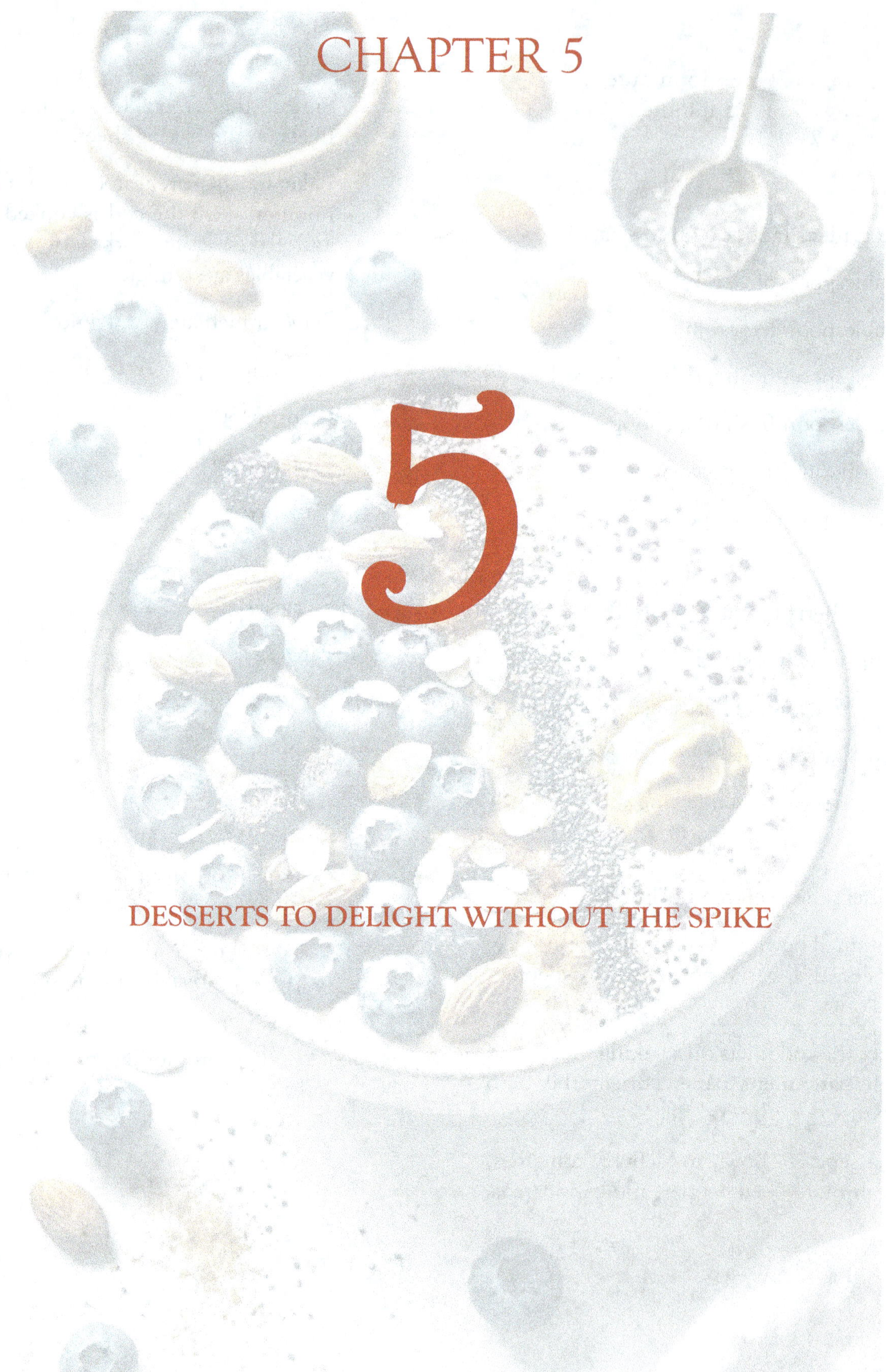

5

DESSERTS TO DELIGHT WITHOUT THE SPIKE

Dark Chocolate Avocado Mousse

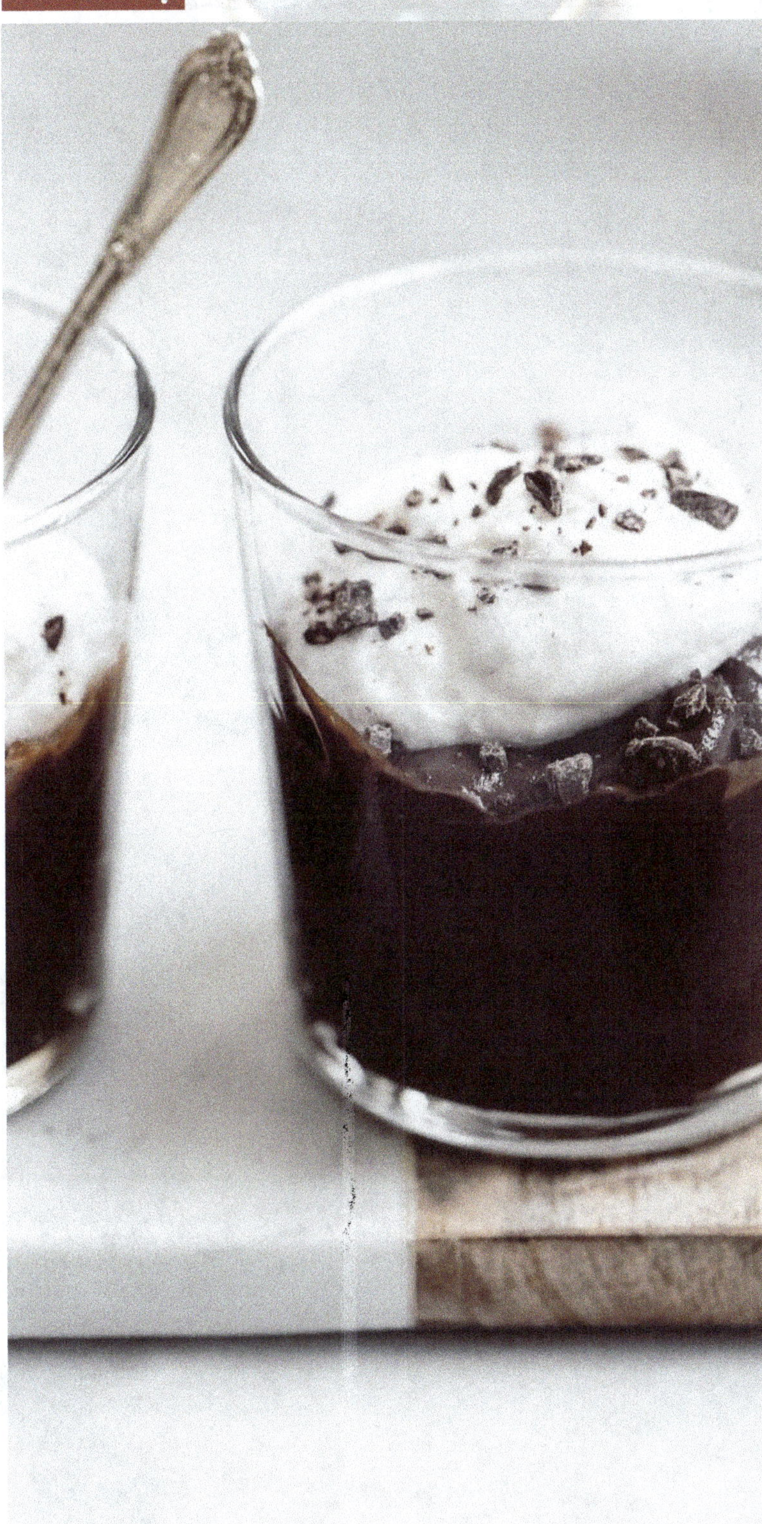

- **Preparation Time:** 10 minutes
- **Cooking Time:** None (Chill for at least 30 minutes)
- **Serving:** 4

Ingredients:

- 2 ripe avocados, peeled and pitted
- 1/4 cup unsweetened cocoa powder
- 1/4 cup almond milk (unsweetened)
- 1/4 cup honey or a few drops of stevia
- 1 teaspoon vanilla extract
- A pinch of salt
- Fresh berries or mint leaves for garnish (optional)

Procedure:

1. In a blender or food processor, combine avocados, cocoa powder, almond milk, honey (or stevia), vanilla extract, and salt.
2. Blend until smooth and creamy, scraping down the sides as needed.
3. Taste and adjust sweetness if necessary.
4. Divide the mousse into four small serving bowls.
5. Chill in the refrigerator for at least 30 minutes before serving.
6. Garnish with fresh berries or mint leaves if desired.
7. Serve and enjoy!

Nutritional Values (per serving):

- Calories: 220
- Protein: 3g
- Carbohydrates: 25g

- Fiber: 7g

- Sugars: 12g (from honey)

- Fat: 14g

- Saturated Fat: 2g

- Sodium: 50mg

Health Benefits:

- **Healthy Fats:** Avocado provides monounsaturated fats that support heart health and satiety.

- **Low Glycemic Index:** The use of stevia or honey in moderation keeps the glycemic index low.

- **High Fiber:** The fiber content helps in maintaining stable blood sugar levels and promoting good digestion.

Berry Chia Pudding

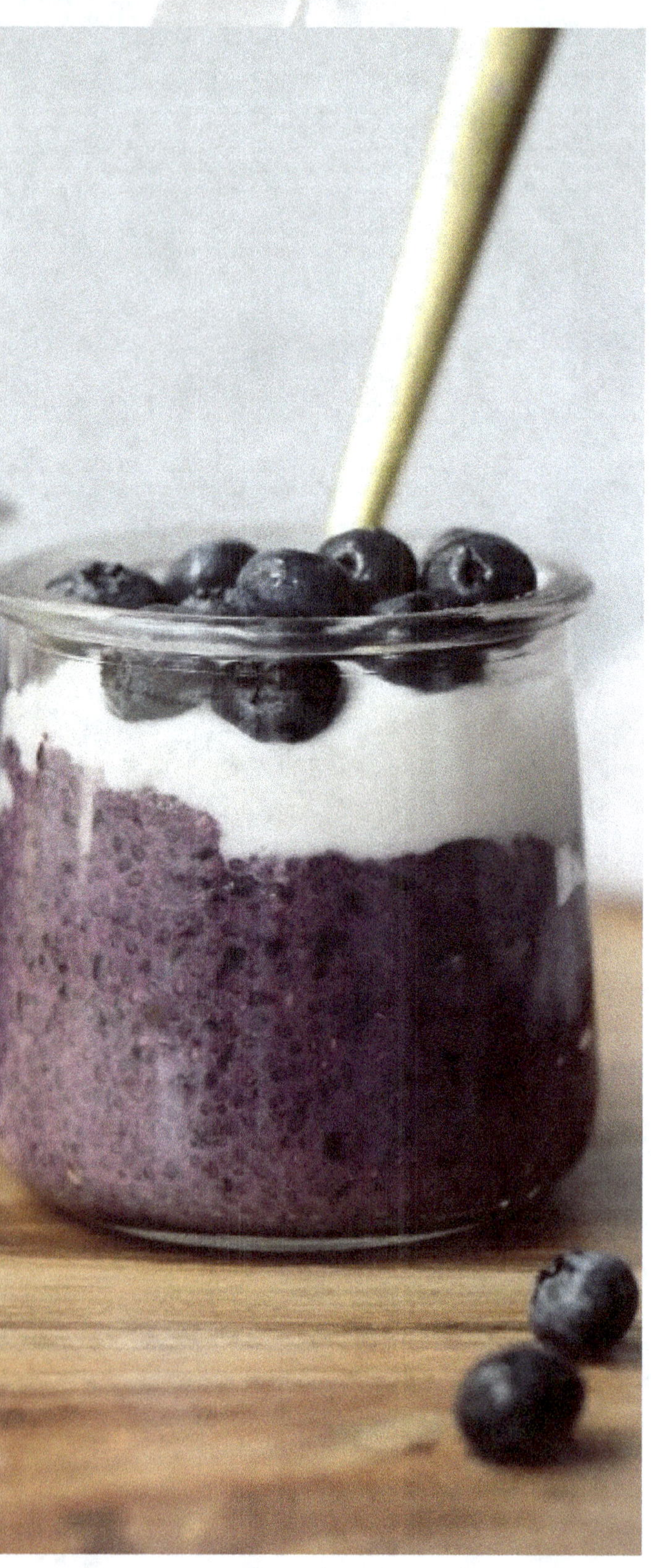

- **Preparation Time:** 10 minutes
- **Cooking Time:** None (Refrigerate overnight)
- **Serving:** 2

Ingredients:

- 1/4 cup chia seeds
- 1 cup unsweetened almond milk
- 1 tablespoon honey or a few drops of stevia
- 1/2 teaspoon vanilla extract
- 1/2 cup mixed berries (blueberries, strawberries, raspberries)
- Fresh mint leaves for garnish (optional)

Procedure:

1. In a medium bowl, whisk together chia seeds, almond milk, honey (or stevia), and vanilla extract.
2. Cover and refrigerate overnight or for at least 4 hours, until the mixture thickens to a pudding-like consistency.
3. Stir the pudding before serving to break up any clumps.
4. Divide the pudding into two serving bowls.
5. Top with mixed berries and garnish with fresh mint leaves if desired.
6. Serve and enjoy!

Nutritional Values (per serving):

- Calories: 180
- Protein: 5g
- Carbohydrates: 20g
- Fiber: 10g
- Sugars: 8g (from honey and berries)
- Fat: 9g
- Saturated Fat: 1g
- Sodium: 50mg

Health Benefits:

- **High Fiber:** Chia seeds and berries provide a substantial amount of fiber, aiding in blood sugar control and digestion.
- **Omega-3 Fatty Acids:** Chia seeds are rich in omega-3s, promoting heart health.
- **Antioxidants:** Berries are packed with antioxidants, supporting overall health and reducing inflammation.

Almond Flour Lemon Bars

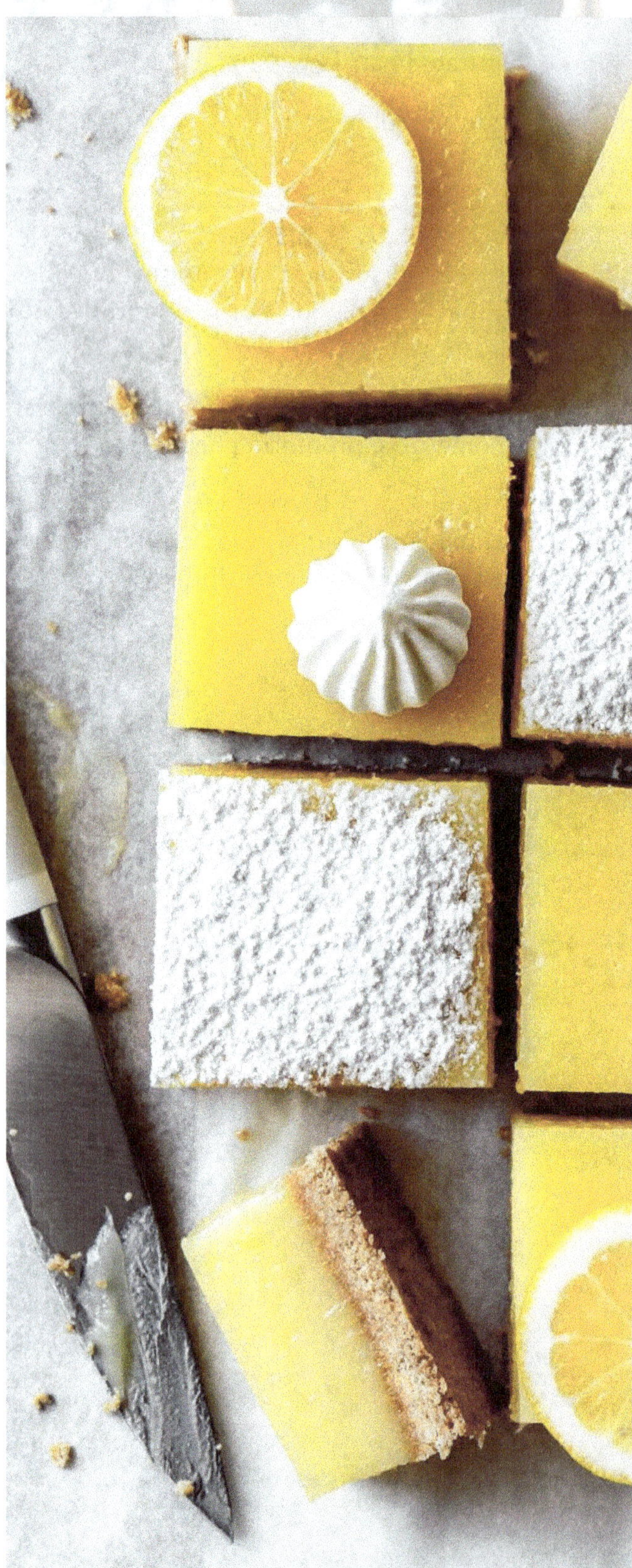

- **Preparation Time:** 15 minutes
- **Cooking Time:** 25 minutes
- **Serving:** 12 bars

Ingredients:

- **For the crust:**
  - 2 cups almond flour
  - 1/4 cup melted coconut oil
  - 1/4 cup honey or a few drops of stevia
  - A pinch of salt
- **For the filling:**
  - 3 large eggs
  - 1/2 cup fresh lemon juice
  - 1/4 cup honey or a few drops of stevia
  - 1 tablespoon lemon zest
  - 2 tablespoons almond flour

Procedure:

1. Preheat the oven to 350°F (175°C).
2. Line an 8x8 inch baking pan with parchment paper.
3. In a medium bowl, mix together almond flour, melted coconut oil, honey (or stevia), and salt until well combined.
4. Press the mixture evenly into the bottom of the prepared baking pan.
5. Bake the crust for 10-12 minutes, until lightly golden.
6. While the crust is baking, prepare the filling. In a large bowl, whisk together eggs, lemon juice, honey (or stevia), lemon zest, and almond flour until smooth.

7. Pour the filling over the pre-baked crust.

8. Bake for an additional 15-18 minutes, until the filling is set and slightly golden around the edges.

9. Allow the bars to cool completely in the pan before cutting into 12 squares.

10. Serve and enjoy!

Nutritional Values (per serving):

- Calories: 150

- Protein: 4g

- Carbohydrates: 10g

- Fiber: 2g

- Sugars: 7g (from honey)

- Fat: 11g

- Saturated Fat: 3g

- Sodium: 45mg

Health Benefits:

- **Low Glycemic Index:** Almond flour and stevia help maintain stable blood sugar levels.

- **Healthy Fats:** Almond flour and coconut oil provide beneficial fats that support heart health and satiety.

- **Rich in Protein:** The bars provide a good source of protein, aiding in muscle maintenance and repair.

Coconut Macaroons

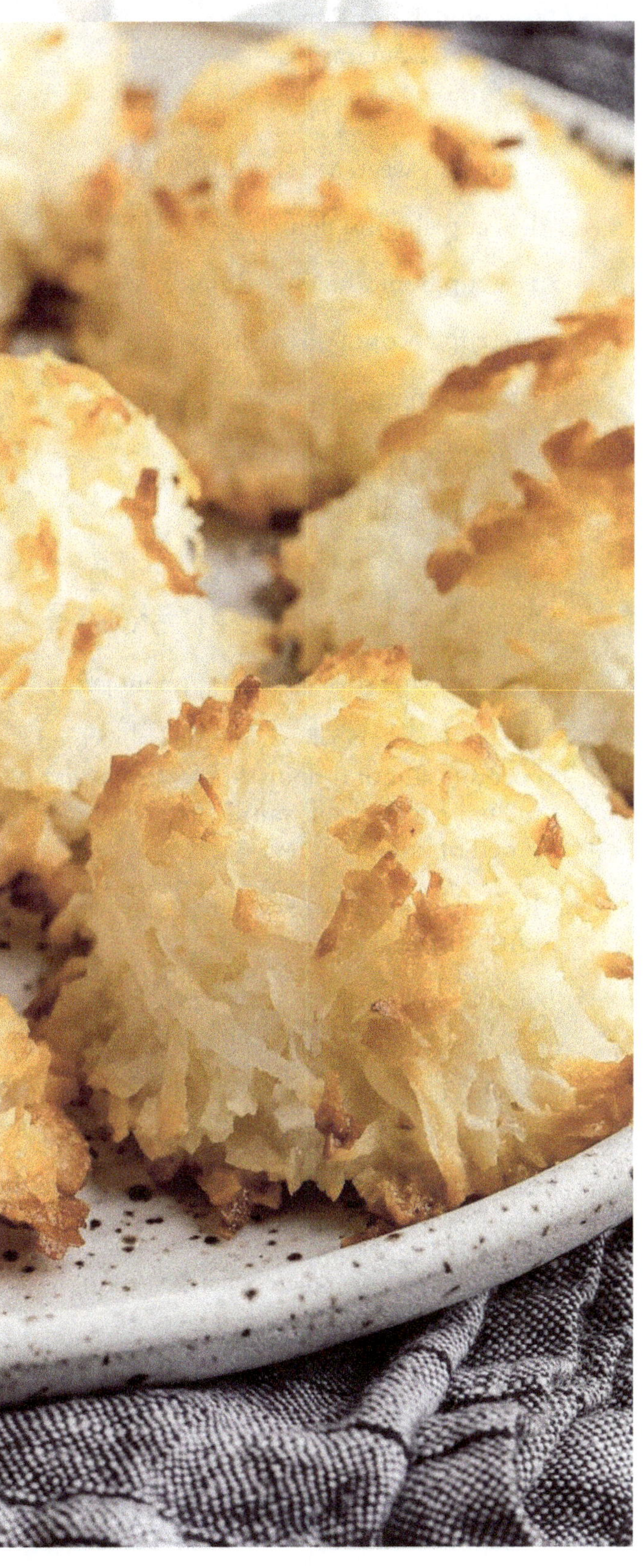

- **Preparation Time:** 10 minutes
- **Cooking Time:** 20 minutes
- **Serving:** 12 macaroons

Ingredients:

- 2 cups unsweetened shredded coconut
- 1/2 cup almond flour
- 1/4 cup honey or a few drops of stevia
- 1/4 cup coconut oil, melted
- 1 teaspoon vanilla extract
- 2 large egg whites
- A pinch of salt

Procedure:

1. Preheat your oven to 350°F (175°C).
2. Line a baking sheet with parchment paper.
3. In a large bowl, combine shredded coconut, almond flour, honey (or stevia), melted coconut oil, vanilla extract, and a pinch of salt.
4. In a separate bowl, beat the egg whites until stiff peaks form.
5. Gently fold the egg whites into the coconut mixture until well combined.
6. Scoop tablespoon-sized mounds of the mixture onto the prepared baking sheet.
7. Bake for 18-20 minutes, until the macaroons are golden brown.
8. Allow to cool completely before serving.
9. Enjoy!

Nutritional Values (per serving):

- Calories: 100
- Protein: 2g
- Carbohydrates: 8g
- Fiber: 3g
- Sugars: 4g (from honey)
- Fat: 8g
- Saturated Fat: 6g
- Sodium: 20mg

Health Benefits:

- **Low Glycemic Index:** Using stevia or a small amount of honey helps keep the glycemic index low, maintaining stable blood sugar levels.
- **Healthy Fats:** Coconut and coconut oil provide medium-chain triglycerides (MCTs), which are beneficial for heart health.
- **High Fiber:** Shredded coconut and almond flour contribute to a high fiber content, aiding in digestion and satiety.

Baked Apples with Cinnamon

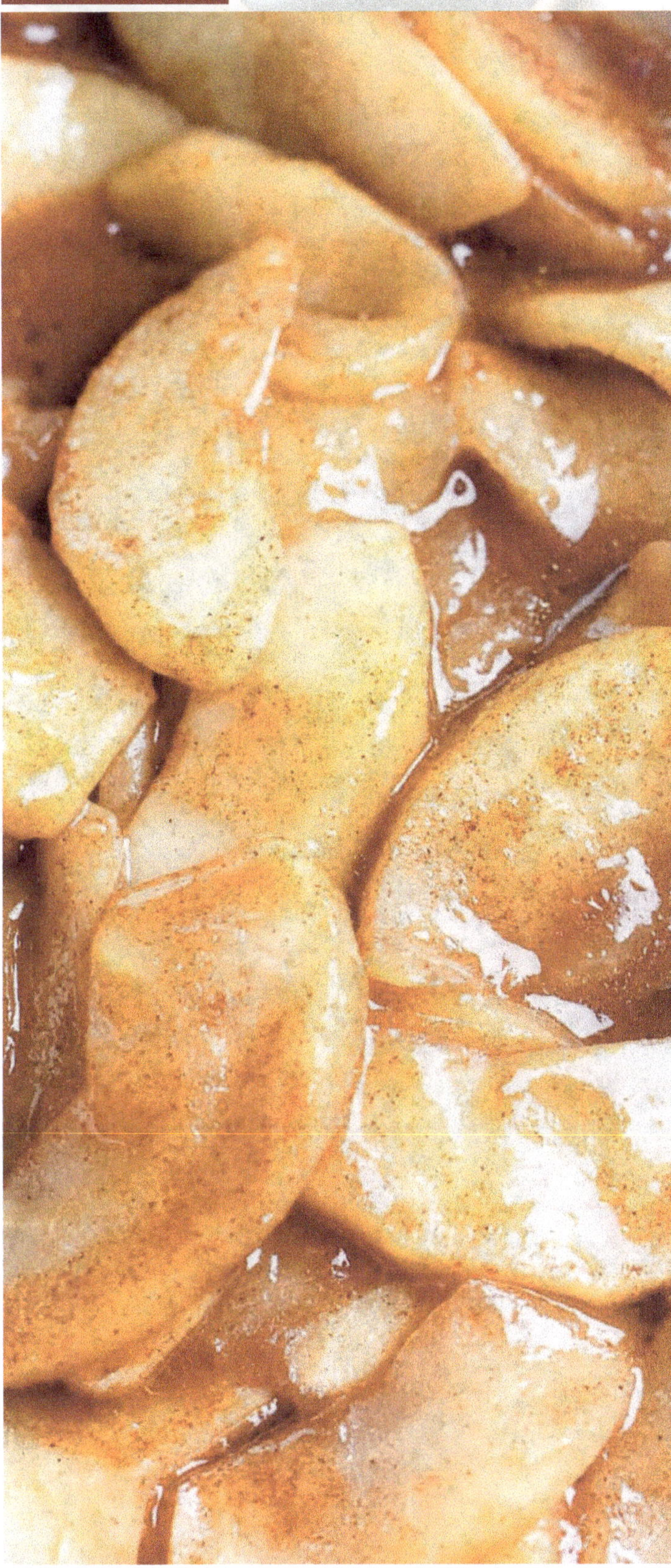

- **Preparation Time:** 10 minutes
- **Cooking Time:** 25 minutes
- **Serving:** 4

Ingredients:

- 4 medium apples, cored and sliced
- 1 tablespoon honey or a few drops of stevia
- 1 teaspoon ground cinnamon
- 1/4 teaspoon ground nutmeg
- 1 tablespoon lemon juice
- 1/4 cup chopped walnuts (optional)

Procedure:

1. Preheat your oven to 375°F (190°C).
2. Place the apple slices in a baking dish.
3. Drizzle with honey (or stevia) and lemon juice.
4. Sprinkle with ground cinnamon and nutmeg.
5. Toss the apples to coat evenly with the mixture.
6. Sprinkle chopped walnuts over the top, if using.
7. Bake for 25 minutes, or until the apples are tender and golden.
8. Serve warm and enjoy!

Nutritional Values (per serving):

- Calories: 120
- Protein: 1g
- Carbohydrates: 28g
- Fiber: 5g
- Sugars: 20g (from apples and honey)

- Fat: 2g

- Saturated Fat: 0.5g

- Sodium: 5mg

Health Benefits:

- **High Fiber:** Apples are rich in fiber, promoting good digestion and prolonged fullness.

- **Antioxidants:** Apples contain antioxidants that support your overall health and reduce inflammation

- **Blood Sugar Management:** The natural sweetness of apples combined with cinnamon helps to regulate blood sugar levels.

Peanut Butter Chocolate Bites

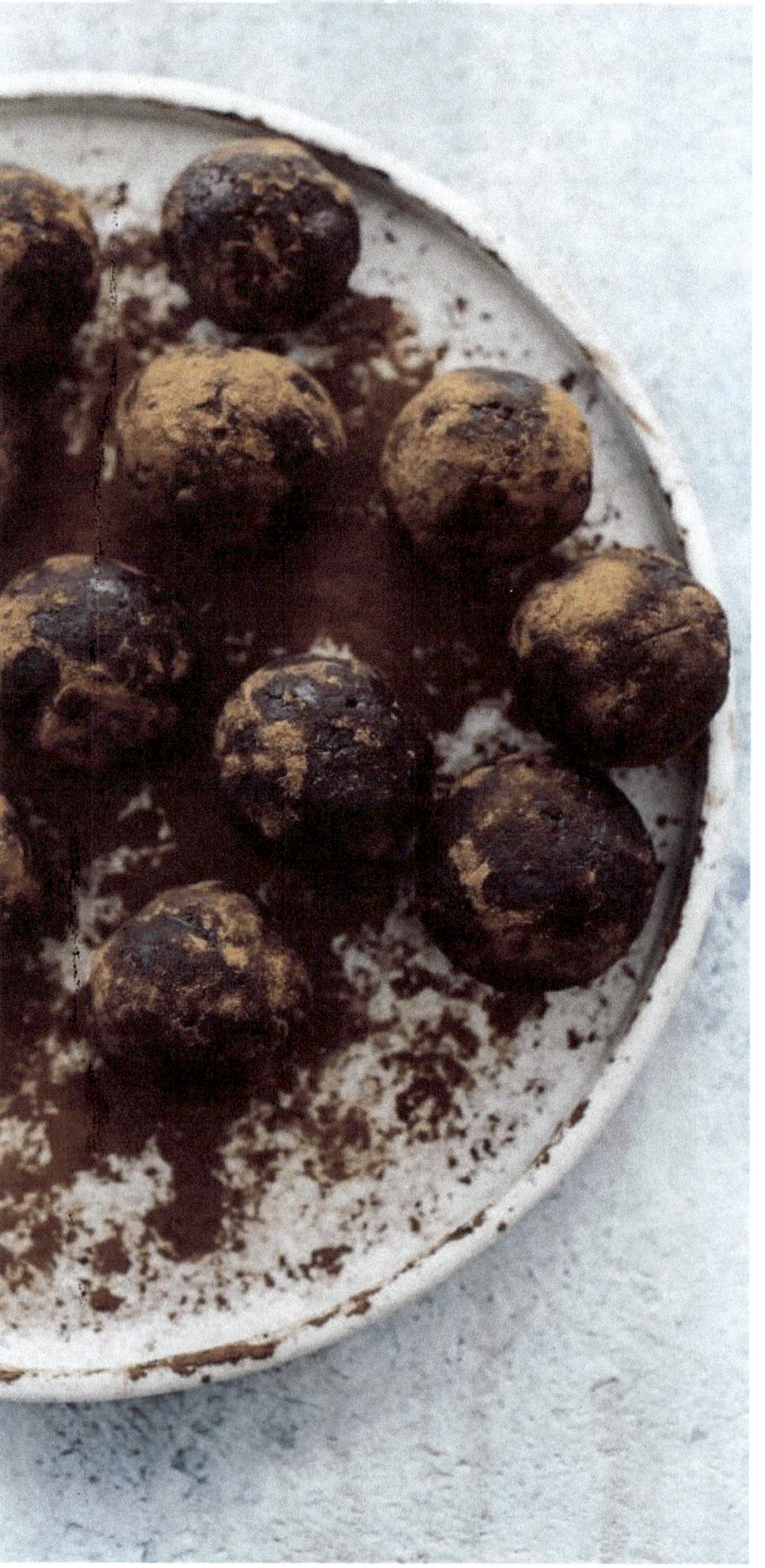

- **Preparation Time:** 10 minutes
- **Cooking Time:** 10 minutes (Chill for 30 minutes)
- **Serving:** 12 bites

Ingredients:

- 1/2 cup natural peanut butter (no added sugar)
- 1/4 cup unsweetened cocoa powder
- 1/4 cup honey or a few drops of stevia
- 1 teaspoon vanilla extract
- 1 cup rolled oats
- 1/4 cup dark chocolate chips (optional)

Procedure:

1. In a medium bowl, combine peanut butter, cocoa powder, honey (or stevia), and vanilla extract. Mix until smooth.
2. Stir in the rolled oats until well combined.
3. If using, fold in dark chocolate chips.
4. Scoop tablespoon-sized portions of the mixture and roll into balls.
5. Place the bites on a baking sheet lined with parchment paper.
6. Chill in the refrigerator for at least 30 minutes before serving.
7. Enjoy!

Nutritional Values (per serving):

- Calories: 120
- Protein: 4g
- Carbohydrates: 14g
- Fiber: 3g
- Sugars: 7g (from honey)
- Fat: 6g
- Saturated Fat: 1.5g
- Sodium: 60mg

Health Benefits:

- **High Protein:** Peanut butter provides protein, essential for muscle maintenance and satiety.
- **Low Glycemic Index:** Using rolled oats and stevia or a small amount of honey helps keep the glycemic index low.
- **Rich in Fiber:** Rolled oats contribute to a high fiber content, aiding in blood sugar control and promoting good digestion.

Sugar-Free Cheesecake Bites

- **Preparation Time:** 15 minutes
- **Cooking Time:** 0 minutes (Chill for at least 1 hour)
- **Serving:** 12 bites

Ingredients:

- 1 cup almond flour
- 1/4 cup melted coconut oil
- 1/4 cup stevia or erythritol
- 1 teaspoon vanilla extract
- 8 ounces cream cheese, softened
- 1/4 cup Greek yogurt (plain, non-fat)
- 1/4 cup stevia or erythritol (for filling)
- 1 teaspoon lemon juice
- Fresh berries for garnish (optional)

Procedure:

1. In a medium bowl, mix almond flour, melted coconut oil, 1/4 cup stevia, and 1/2 teaspoon vanilla extract until well combined.

2. Press the mixture evenly into the bottom of a mini muffin tin lined with paper liners to form the crust.

3. In another bowl, beat the softened cream cheese until smooth.

4. Add Greek yogurt, 1/4 cup stevia, 1/2 teaspoon vanilla extract, and lemon juice to the cream cheese and mix until creamy and well combined.

5. Spoon the cream cheese mixture over the crust in the muffin tin, filling each cup.

6. Smooth the tops with a spoon or spatula.

7. Chill in the refrigerator for at least 1 hour to set.

8. Garnish with fresh berries if desired before serving.

9. Enjoy!

Nutritional Values (per serving):

- Calories: 120

- Protein: 3g

- Carbohydrates: 5g

- Fiber: 1g

- Sugars: 1g (from berries, if used)

- Fat: 10g

- Saturated Fat: 5g

- Sodium: 70mg

Health Benefits:

- **Low Glycemic Index:** Using stevia or erythritol keeps the glycemic index low, maintaining stable blood sugar levels.

- **High Protein:** Greek yogurt and cream cheese provide protein, essential for muscle maintenance and satiety.

- **Healthy Fats:** Almond flour and coconut oil contribute beneficial fats that support heart health.

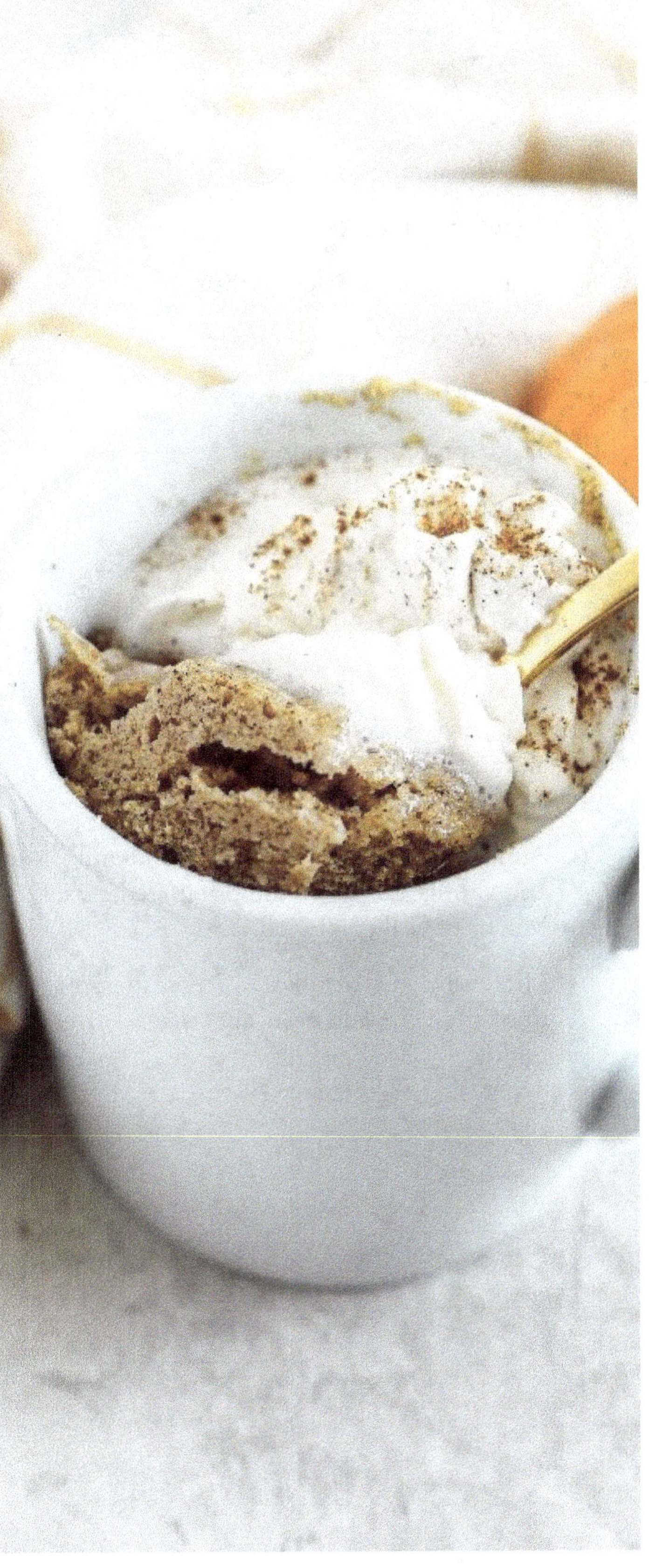

- **Preparation Time:** 5 minutes
- **Cooking Time:** 2 minutes
- **Serving:** 1

Ingredients:

- 1/4 cup almond flour
- 1 tablespoon coconut flour
- 1 tablespoon stevia or erythritol
- 1/4 teaspoon baking powder
- 1/4 teaspoon pumpkin pie spice
- 1/4 cup pumpkin puree
- 1 large egg
- 1 tablespoon unsweetened almond milk
- 1/2 teaspoon vanilla extract

Procedure:

1. In a microwave-safe mug, whisk together almond flour, coconut flour, stevia, baking powder, and pumpkin pie spice.

2. Add pumpkin puree, egg, almond milk, and vanilla extract to the dry ingredients. Mix until well combined.

3. Microwave on high for 1-2 minutes, or until the cake has risen and is set in the middle. Cooking time may vary depending on the microwave.

4. Allow the mug cake to cool for a minute before enjoying.

5. Serve and enjoy!

Nutritional Values (per serving):

- Calories: 180
- Protein: 8g
- Carbohydrates: 10g
- Fiber: 5g
- Sugars: 3g
- Fat: 12g
- Saturated Fat: 3g
- Sodium: 150mg

Health Benefits:

- **Low Glycemic Index:** Almond flour and stevia help keep the glycemic index low, supporting stable blood sugar levels.

- **High Fiber:** Coconut flour and pumpkin puree contribute to a high fiber content, promoting good digestion and satiety.

- **Protein-Packed:** The egg provides essential protein for muscle maintenance and repair.

CHAPTER 6

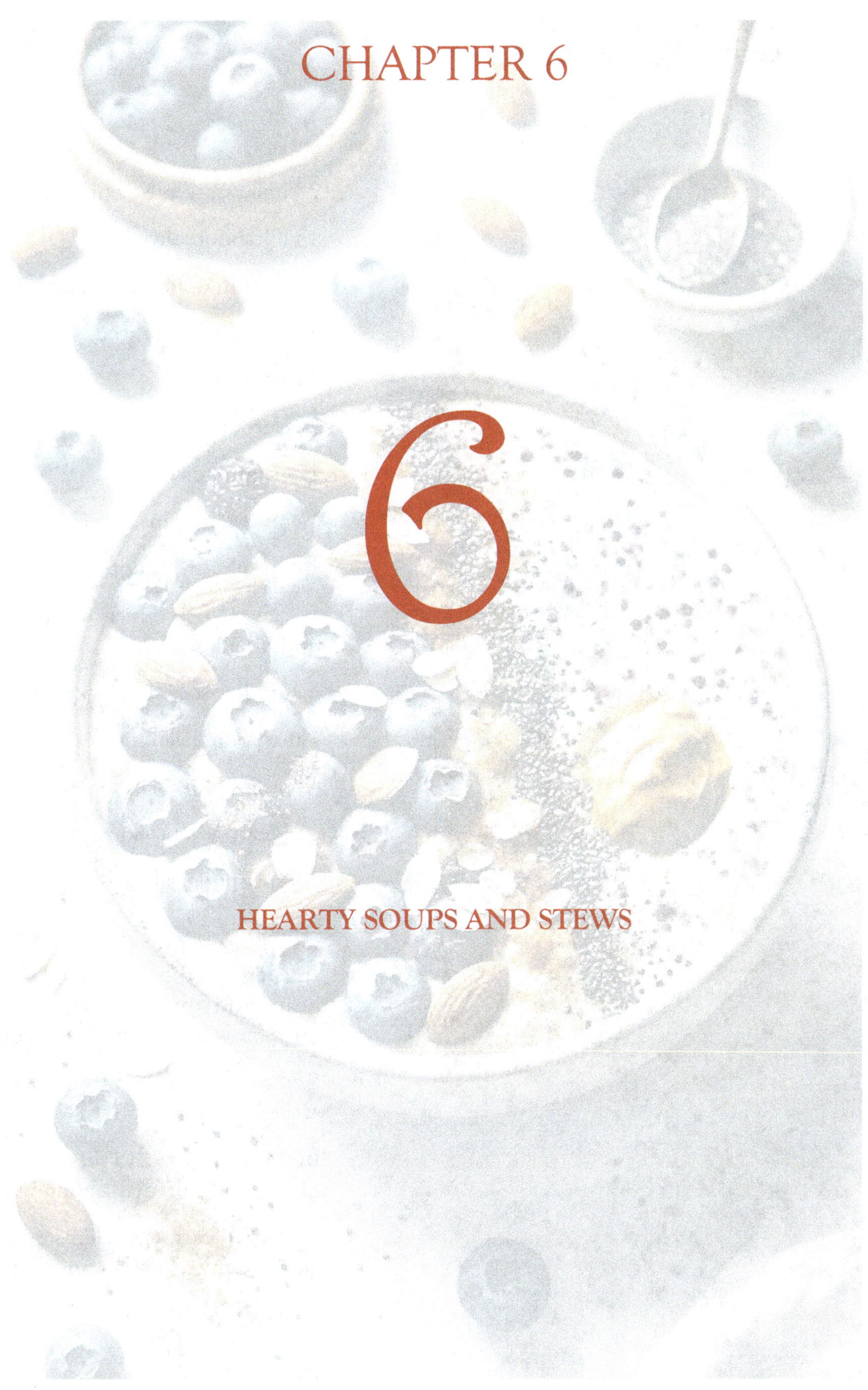

HEARTY SOUPS AND STEWS

Hearty Chicken Vegetable Soup

- **Preparation Time:** 15 minutes
- **Cooking Time:** 45 minutes
- **Serving:** 4

Ingredients:

- 2 boneless, skinless chicken breasts, diced
- 1 tablespoon olive oil
- 1 medium onion, chopped
- 2 cloves garlic, minced
- 2 carrots, sliced
- 2 celery stalks, sliced
- 1 zucchini, diced
- 1 cup green beans, cut into 1-inch pieces
- 1 cup spinach, chopped
- 1 can (14.5 ounces) diced tomatoes, undrained
- 6 cups low-sodium chicken broth
- 1 teaspoon dried thyme
- 1 teaspoon dried basil
- 1/4 teaspoon black pepper
- 1/4 teaspoon salt

Procedure:

1. In a large pot, heat olive oil over medium heat. Add the diced chicken and cook until browned, about 5-7 minutes.

2. Remove the chicken from the pot and set aside.

3. In the same pot, add the onion and garlic. Sauté until softened, about 3 minutes.

4. Add the carrots, celery, zucchini, and green beans. Cook for another 5 minutes, stirring occasionally.

5. Pour in the diced tomatoes and chicken broth. Stir in thyme, basil, black pepper, and salt.

6. Return the chicken to the pot. Bring to a boil, then reduce the heat and let it simmer for 30 minutes.

7. Add the chopped spinach and cook for another 5 minutes until wilted.

8. Serve hot and enjoy!

Nutritional Values (per serving):

- Calories: 200

- Protein: 22g

- Carbohydrates: 18g

- Fiber: 5g

- Sugars: 7g

- Fat: 6g

- Saturated Fat: 1g

- Sodium: 350mg

Health Benefits:

- **High Protein:** Chicken provides essential protein for muscle maintenance and satiety.

- **Low Glycemic Index:** Vegetables and chicken help maintain stable blood sugar levels.

- **Rich in Fiber:** Vegetables add fiber, aiding digestion and promoting fullness.

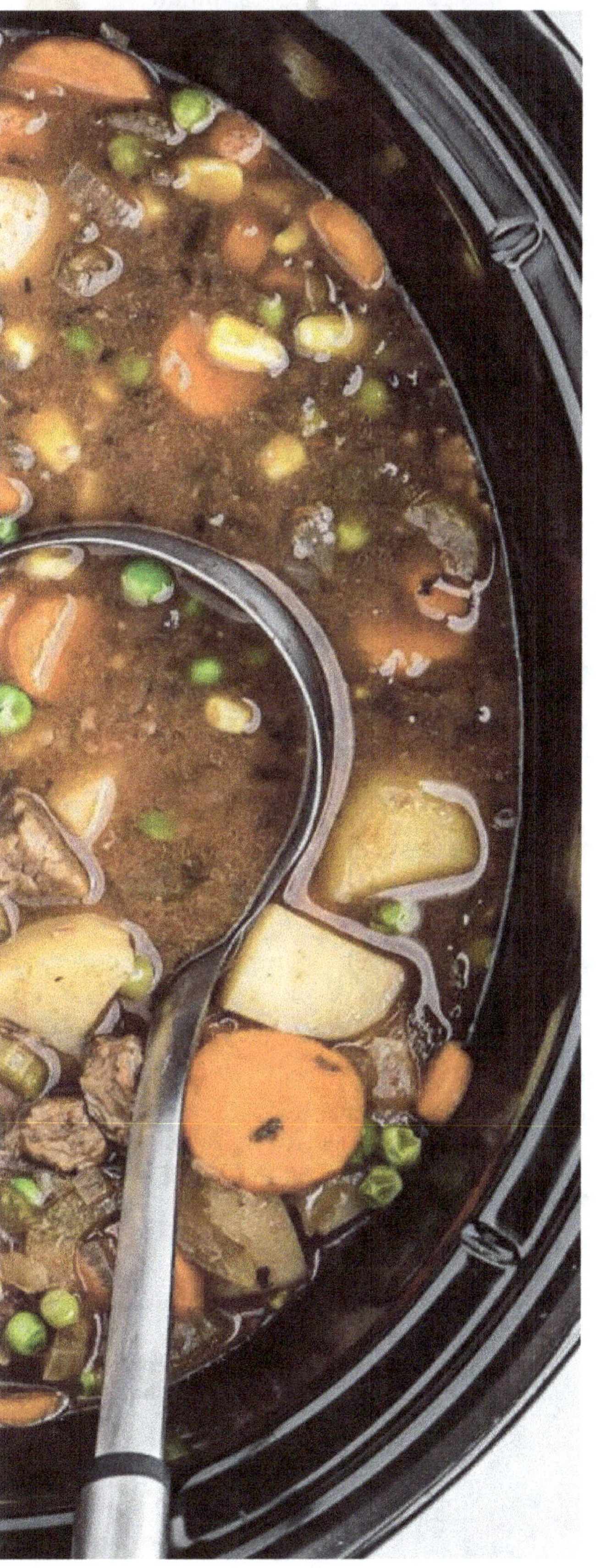

- **Preparation Time:** 15 minutes
- **Cooking Time:** 6-8 hours (slow cooker)
- **Serving:** 6

Ingredients:

- 1 1/2 pounds lean beef stew meat, cut into 1-inch cubes
- 2 tablespoons olive oil
- 4 carrots, sliced
- 3 celery stalks, sliced
- 3 potatoes, diced
- 1 large onion, chopped
- 3 cloves garlic, minced
- 1 can (14.5 ounces) diced tomatoes, undrained
- 4 cups low-sodium beef broth
- 1 teaspoon dried thyme
- 1 teaspoon dried rosemary
- 1/4 teaspoon black pepper
- 1/4 teaspoon salt
- 2 tablespoons cornstarch mixed with 2 tablespoons water (optional, for thickening)

Procedure:

1. Heat olive oil in a large skillet over medium-high heat. Add the beef and cook until browned on all sides, about 5-7 minutes.
2. Transfer the beef to a slow cooker.
3. Add the carrots, celery, potatoes, onion, and garlic to the slow cooker.
4. Pour in the diced tomatoes and beef broth. Stir in thyme, rosemary, black pepper, and salt.
5. Cover and cook on low for 6-8 hours, or until the beef and vegetables are tender.
6. If you prefer a thicker stew, mix the cornstarch and water, then stir it into the stew during the last 30 minutes of cooking.
7. Serve hot and enjoy!

Nutritional Values (per serving):

- Calories: 300
- Protein: 30g
- Carbohydrates: 25g
- Fiber: 5g
- Sugars: 6g
- Fat: 10g
- Saturated Fat: 3g
- Sodium: 400mg

Health Benefits:

- **High Protein:** Lean beef provides essential protein for muscle health and satiety.
- **Rich in Fiber:** Vegetables add fiber, promoting good digestion and fullness.
- **Low Glycemic Index:** Helps maintain stable blood sugar levels.

Creamy Cauliflower Soup

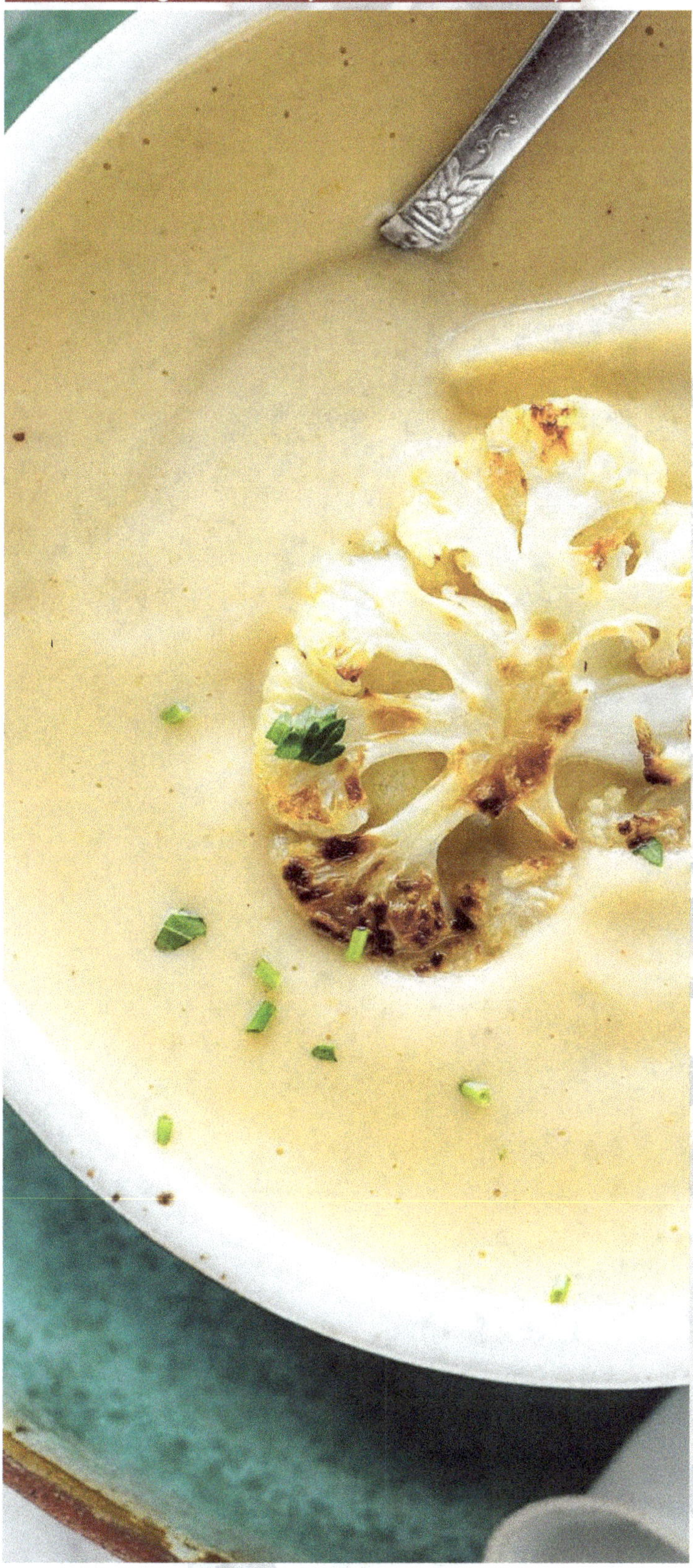

- **Preparation Time:** 10 minutes
- **Cooking Time:** 25 minutes
- **Serving:** 4

Ingredients:

- 1 large head cauliflower, chopped
- 1 tablespoon olive oil
- 1 medium onion, chopped
- 2 cloves garlic, minced
- 4 cups low-sodium vegetable broth
- 1 cup unsweetened almond milk
- 1 teaspoon dried thyme
- 1/4 teaspoon black pepper
- 1/4 teaspoon salt
- Fresh chives for garnish (optional)

Procedure:

1. In a large pot, heat olive oil over medium heat. Add the onion and garlic, and sauté until softened, about 3 minutes.

2. Add the chopped cauliflower and cook for another 5 minutes, stirring occasionally.

3. Pour in the vegetable broth and bring to a boil. Reduce the heat and let it simmer for 15 minutes, until the cauliflower is tender.

4. Using an immersion blender, puree the soup until smooth. Alternatively, transfer the soup in batches to a blender and puree.

5. Stir in the almond milk, thyme, black pepper, and salt. Cook for another 2 minutes until heated through.

6. Garnish with fresh chives if desired.

7. Serve hot and enjoy!

Nutritional Values (per serving):

- Calories: 100

- Protein: 4g

- Carbohydrates: 12g

- Fiber: 4g

- Sugars: 4g

- Fat: 4g

- Saturated Fat: 0.5g

- Sodium: 250mg

Health Benefits:

- **Low Glycemic Index:** Cauliflower and almond milk help maintain stable blood sugar levels.

- **High Fiber:** Cauliflower provides fiber, aiding digestion and promoting fullness.

- **Low Calorie:** A light yet satisfying option for maintaining a healthy weight.

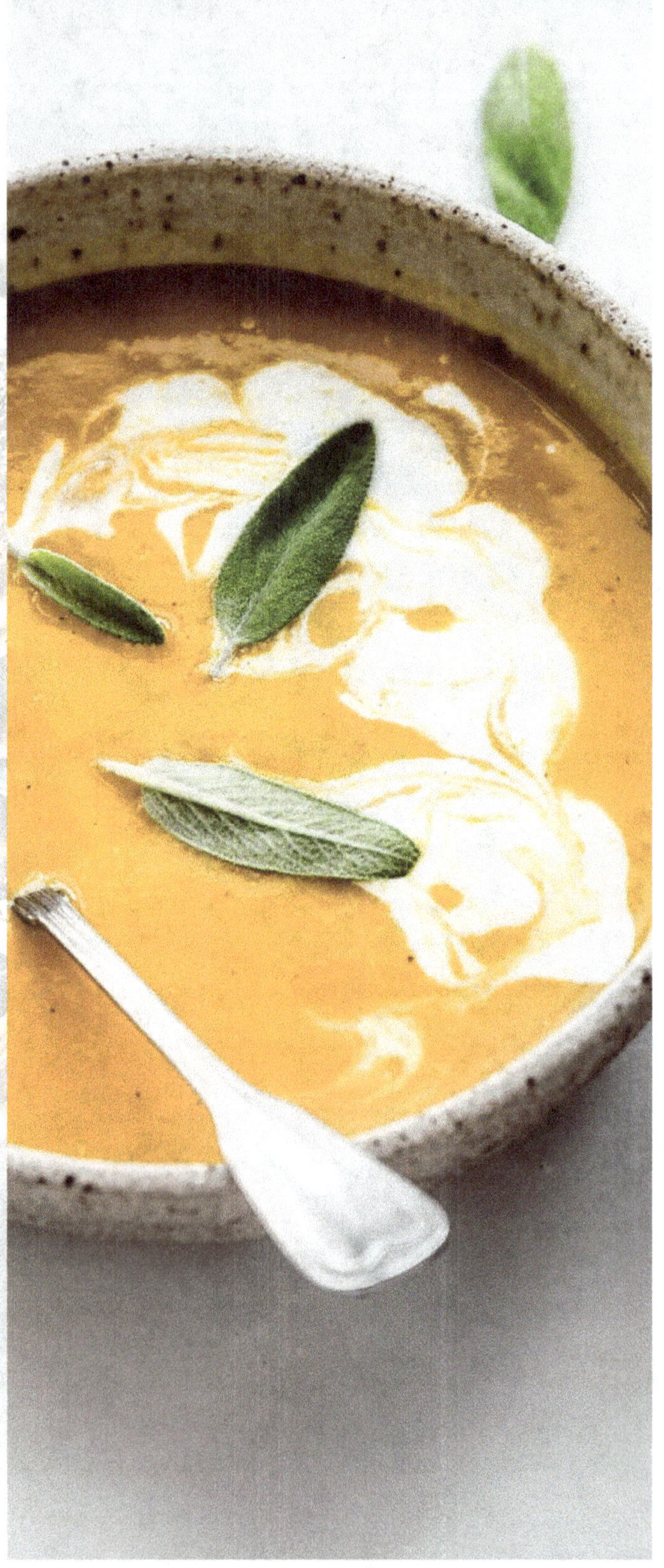

- **Preparation Time:** 15 minutes
- **Cooking Time:** 30 minutes
- **Serving:** 4

Ingredients:

- 1 medium butternut squash, peeled, seeded, and cubed

- 2 apples, peeled, cored, and chopped

- 1 tablespoon olive oil

- 1 medium onion, chopped

- 2 cloves garlic, minced

- 4 cups low-sodium vegetable broth

- 1 teaspoon ground cinnamon

- 1/2 teaspoon ground nutmeg

- 1/4 teaspoon black pepper

- 1/4 teaspoon salt

Procedure:

1. In a large pot, heat olive oil over medium heat. Add the onion and garlic, and sauté until softened, about 3 minutes.

2. Add the butternut squash and apples, and cook for another 5 minutes, stirring occasionally.

3. Pour in the vegetable broth and bring to a boil. Reduce the heat and let it simmer for 20 minutes, until the squash and apples are tender.

4. Using an immersion blender, puree the soup until smooth. Alternatively, transfer the soup in batches to a blender and puree.

5. Stir in the cinnamon, nutmeg, black pepper, and salt. Cook for another 2 minutes until heated through.

6. Serve hot and enjoy!

Nutritional Values (per serving):

- Calories: 150

- Protein: 2g

- Carbohydrates: 30g

- Fiber: 5g

- Sugars: 12g

- Fat: 4g

- Saturated Fat: 0.5g

- Sodium: 250mg

Health Benefits:

- **High Fiber:** Butternut squash and apples provide fiber, aiding digestion and promoting fullness.

- **Antioxidants:** Squash and apples are rich in antioxidants, supporting overall health and reducing inflammation.

- **Low Glycemic Index:** Helps maintain stable blood sugar levels.

CHAPTER 7

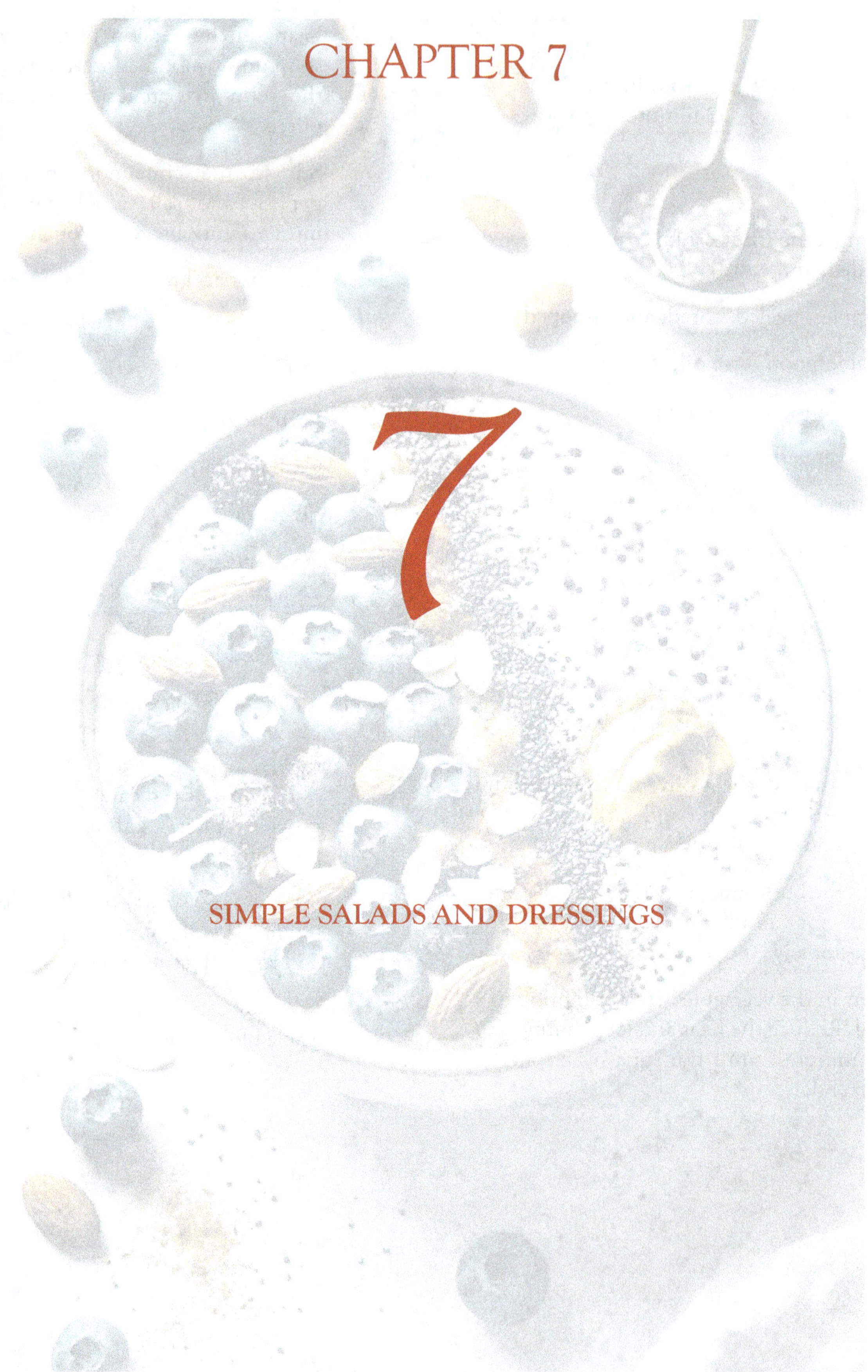

SIMPLE SALADS AND DRESSINGS

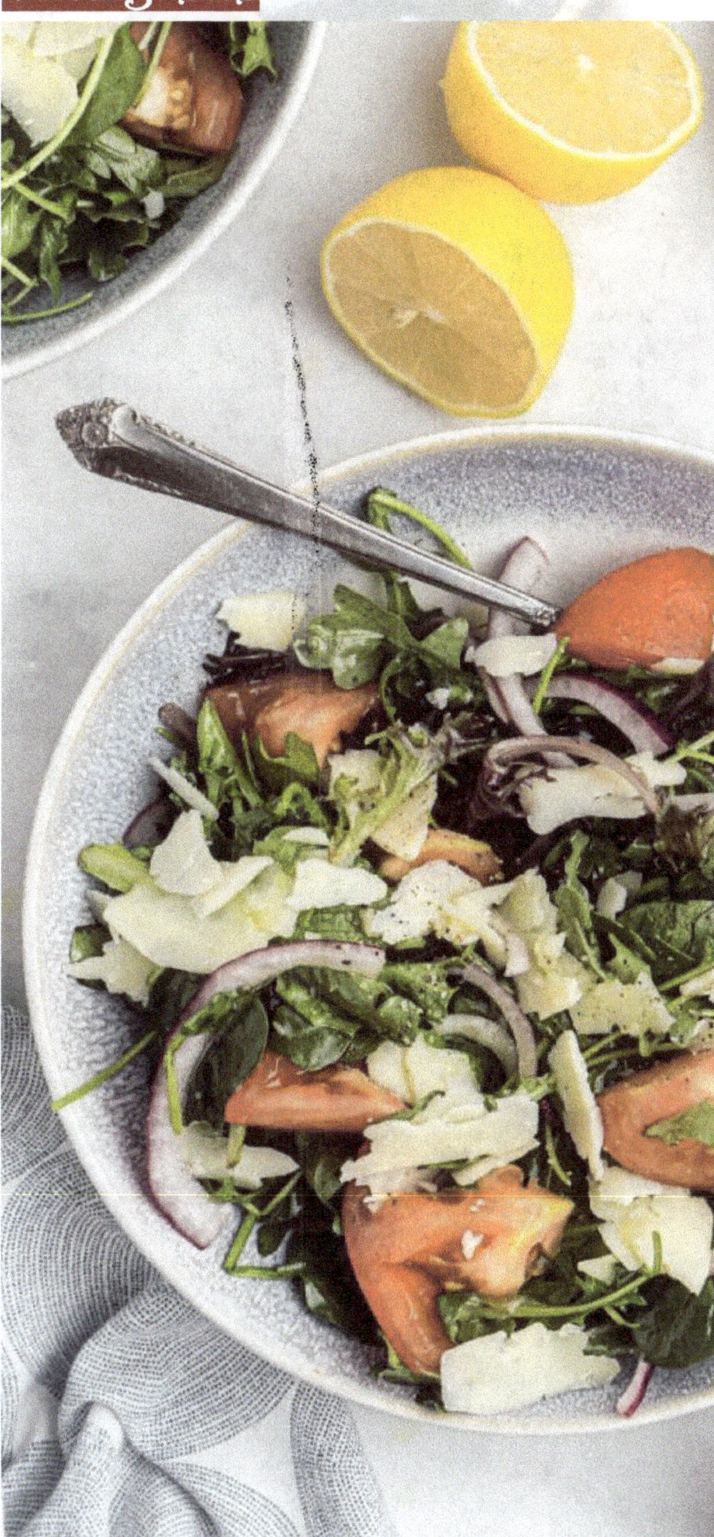

- **Preparation Time:** 10 minutes
- **Cooking Time:** None
- **Serving:** 4

Ingredients:

- 4 cups mixed greens (such as arugula, spinach, and lettuce)
- 1/4 cup extra-virgin olive oil
- 2 tablespoons fresh lemon juice
- 1 teaspoon Dijon mustard
- 1 teaspoon honey or a few drops of stevia
- 1/4 teaspoon black pepper
- 1/4 teaspoon salt

Procedure:

1. In a small bowl, whisk together olive oil, lemon juice, Dijon mustard, honey (or stevia), black pepper, and salt until well combined.
2. Place the mixed greens in a large salad bowl.
3. Drizzle the lemon vinaigrette over the greens and toss gently to coat.
4. Serve immediately and enjoy!

Nutritional Values (per serving):

- Calories: 100
- Protein: 1g
- Carbohydrates: 3g
- Fiber: 2g
- Sugars: 1g (from honey)
- Fat: 9g
- Saturated Fat: 1g
- Sodium: 150mg

Health Benefits:

- **Low Glycemic Index:** Helps maintain stable blood sugar levels.

- **Healthy Fats:** Olive oil provides heart-healthy monounsaturated fats.

- **Rich in Fiber:** Mixed greens offer fiber, aiding digestion and promoting fullness.

Cucumber and Tomato Salad with Feta

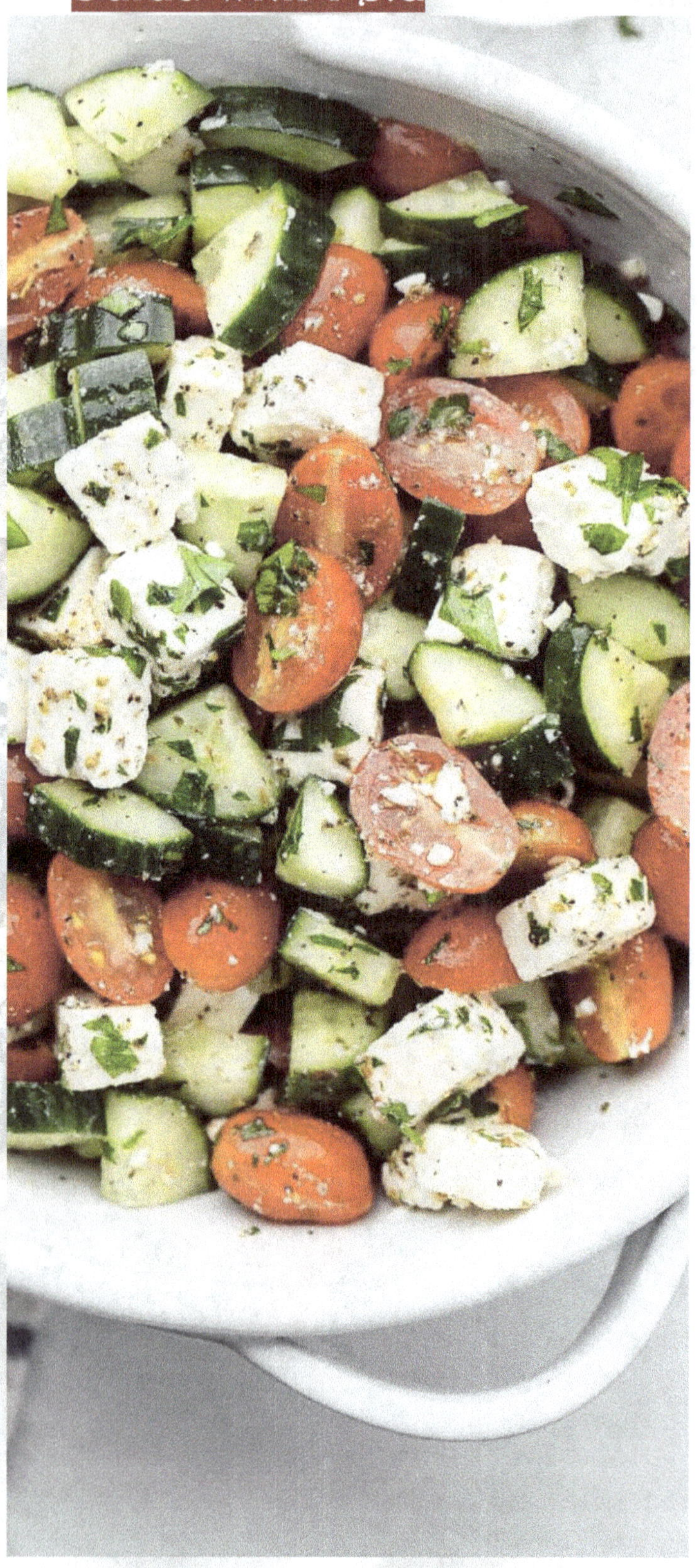

- **Preparation Time:** 10 minutes
- **Cooking Time:** None
- **Serving:** 4

Ingredients:

- 2 cups cucumber, diced

- 2 cups cherry tomatoes, halved

- 1/4 cup red onion, finely chopped

- 1/4 cup feta cheese, crumbled

- 2 tablespoons olive oil

- 1 tablespoon red wine vinegar

- 1 teaspoon dried oregano

- 1/4 teaspoon black pepper

- 1/4 teaspoon salt

Procedure:

1. In a large bowl, combine cucumber, cherry tomatoes, red onion, and feta cheese.

2. In a small bowl, whisk together olive oil, red wine vinegar, oregano, black pepper, and salt.

3. Pour the dressing over the salad and toss gently to combine.

4. Serve immediately and enjoy!

Nutritional Values (per serving):

- Calories: 120

- Protein: 3g

- Carbohydrates: 6g

- Fiber: 2g

- Sugars: 3g

- Fat: 10g

- Saturated Fat: 3g

- Sodium: 250mg

Health Benefits:

- **Low Glycemic Index:** Helps maintain stable blood sugar levels.

- **Healthy Fats:** Olive oil provides monounsaturated fats that support heart health.

- **Antioxidants:** Tomatoes and cucumbers are rich in antioxidants, promoting overall health.

Kale and Quinoa Salad

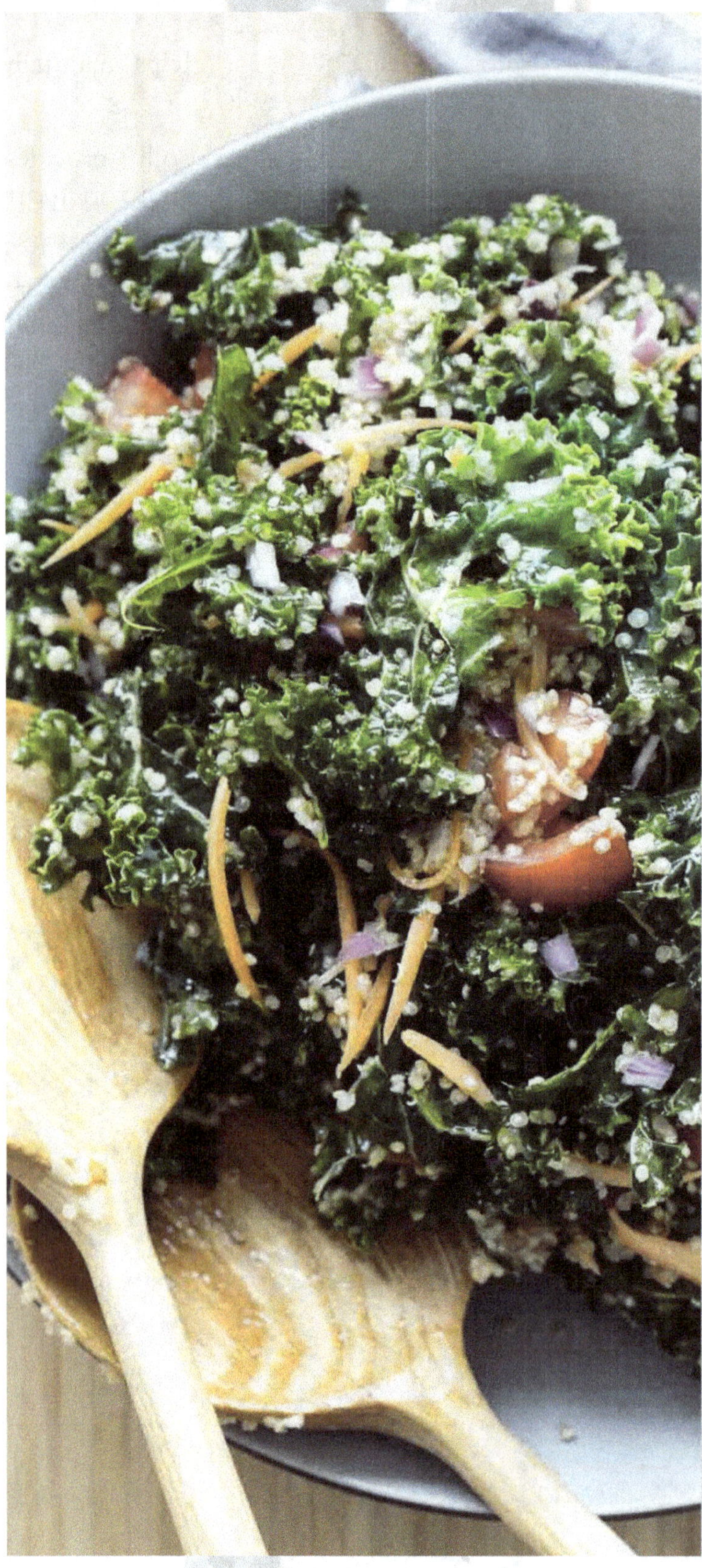

- **Preparation Time:** 15 minutes
- **Cooking Time:** 15 minutes
- **Serving:** 4

Ingredients:

- 1 cup quinoa
- 2 cups water
- 4 cups kale, chopped
- 1/2 cup red bell pepper, diced
- 1/2 cup shredded carrots
- 1/4 cup sunflower seeds
- 1/4 cup dried cranberries (unsweetened)
- 1/4 cup olive oil
- 2 tablespoons apple cider vinegar
- 1 tablespoon lemon juice
- 1 teaspoon Dijon mustard
- 1/4 teaspoon black pepper
- 1/4 teaspoon salt

Procedure:

1. Rinse quinoa under cold water.

2. In a medium saucepan, bring quinoa and water to a boil. Reduce heat, cover, and simmer for about 15 minutes, or until water is absorbed and quinoa is tender.

3. In a large bowl, combine cooked quinoa, kale, red bell pepper, shredded carrots, sunflower seeds, and dried cranberries.

4. In a small bowl, whisk together olive oil, apple cider vinegar, lemon juice, Dijon mustard, black pepper, and salt.

5. Pour the dressing over the salad and toss gently to combine.

6. Serve immediately or chill in the refrigerator for enhanced flavors.

7. Enjoy!

Nutritional Values (per serving):

- Calories: 250

- Protein: 6g

- Carbohydrates: 30g

- Fiber: 5g

- Sugars: 6g

- Fat: 12g

- Saturated Fat: 1.5g

- Sodium: 200mg

Health Benefits:

- **High Fiber:** Quinoa and kale provide substantial fiber, aiding digestion and promoting satiety.

- **Low Glycemic Index:** Helps maintain stable blood sugar levels.

- **Nutrient-Dense:** Kale and quinoa are rich in vitamins, minerals, and antioxidants, supporting overall health.

Spinach and Strawberry Salad

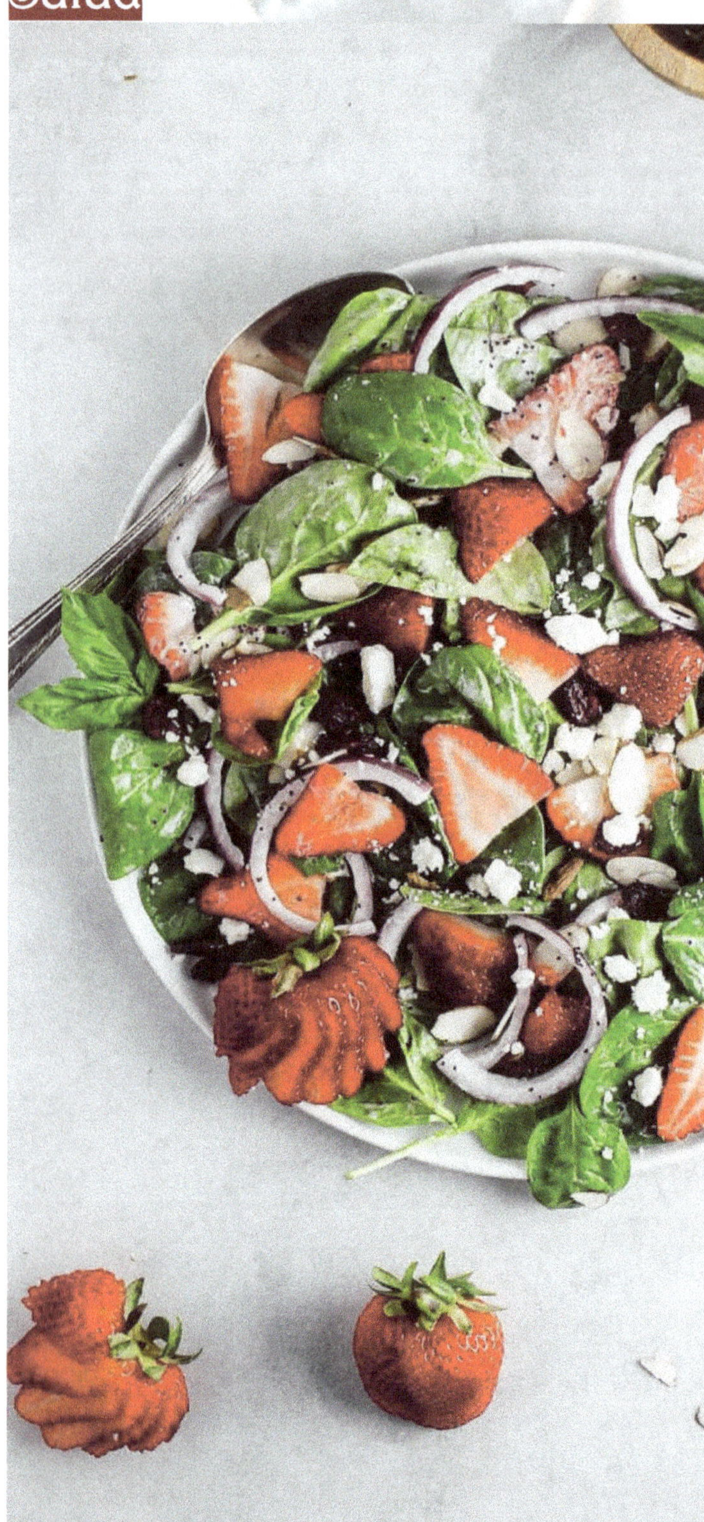

- **Preparation Time:** 10 minutes
- **Cooking Time:** None
- **Serving:** 4

Ingredients:

- 4 cups fresh spinach leaves
- 1 cup strawberries, sliced
- 1/4 cup red onion, thinly sliced
- 1/4 cup sliced almonds
- 2 tablespoons olive oil
- 1 tablespoon balsamic vinegar
- 1 teaspoon honey or a few drops of stevia
- 1/4 teaspoon black pepper
- 1/4 teaspoon salt

Procedure:

1. In a large salad bowl, combine spinach, strawberries, red onion, and sliced almonds.

2. In a small bowl, whisk together olive oil, balsamic vinegar, honey (or stevia), black pepper, and salt.

3. Drizzle the dressing over the salad and toss gently to coat.

4. Serve immediately and enjoy!

Nutritional Values (per serving):

- Calories: 130
- Protein: 3g
- Carbohydrates: 10g
- Fiber: 3g
- Sugars: 6g (from strawberries)
- Fat: 9g
- Saturated Fat: 1g

- Sodium: 100mg

Health Benefits:

- **Low Glycemic Index:** Helps maintain stable blood sugar levels.

- **High Fiber:** Spinach and strawberries provide fiber, aiding digestion and promoting fullness.

- **Antioxidants:** Strawberries and spinach are rich in antioxidants, supporting overall health and reducing inflammation.

Roasted Beet and Goat Cheese Salad

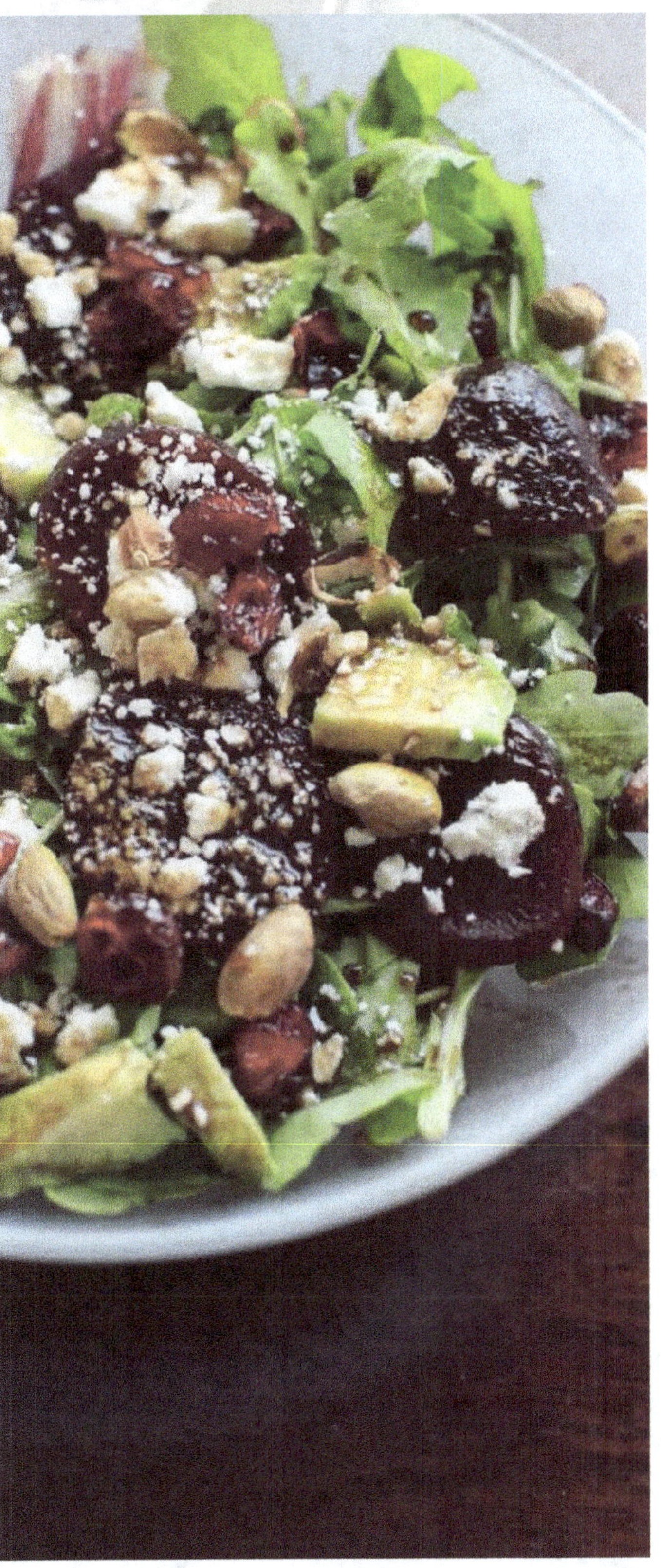

- **Preparation Time:** 15 minutes
- **Cooking Time:** 40 minutes
- **Serving:** 4

Ingredients:

- 4 medium beets, roasted and diced

- 4 cups mixed greens (such as arugula, spinach, and lettuce)

- 1/4 cup goat cheese, crumbled

- 1/4 cup walnuts, chopped

- 2 tablespoons olive oil

- 1 tablespoon balsamic vinegar

- 1 teaspoon Dijon mustard

- 1/4 teaspoon black pepper

- 1/4 teaspoon salt

Procedure:

1. Preheat your oven to 400°F (200°C).

2. Wrap each beet in foil and roast in the preheated oven for about 40 minutes, or until tender.

3. Allow the beets to cool, then peel and dice them.

4. In a large salad bowl, combine mixed greens, diced beets, goat cheese, and chopped walnuts.

5. In a small bowl, whisk together olive oil, balsamic vinegar, Dijon mustard, black pepper, and salt.

6. Drizzle the dressing over the salad and toss gently to coat.

7. Serve immediately and enjoy!

Nutritional Values (per serving):

- Calories: 180

- Protein: 4g

- Carbohydrates: 16g

- Fiber: 5g

- Sugars: 8g (from beets)

- Fat: 12g

- Saturated Fat: 3g

- Sodium: 250mg

Health Benefits:

- **Low Glycemic Index:** Beets and mixed greens help maintain stable blood sugar levels.

- **Rich in Fiber:** Beets and greens provide substantial fiber, aiding digestion and promoting fullness.

- **Healthy Fats:** Olive oil and walnuts contribute beneficial fats that support heart health.

CHAPTER 8

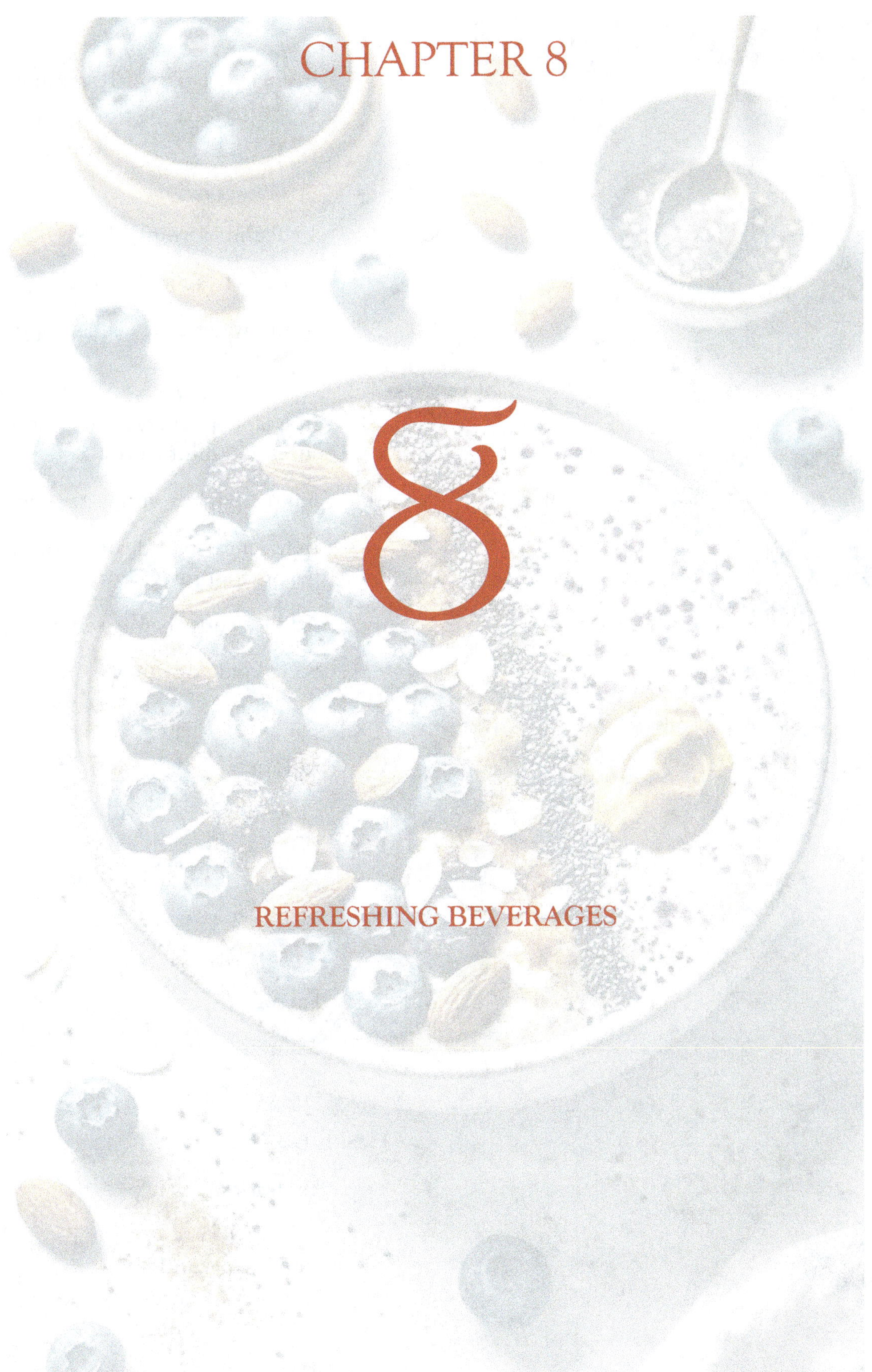

REFRESHING BEVERAGES

Cucumber Mint Infused Water

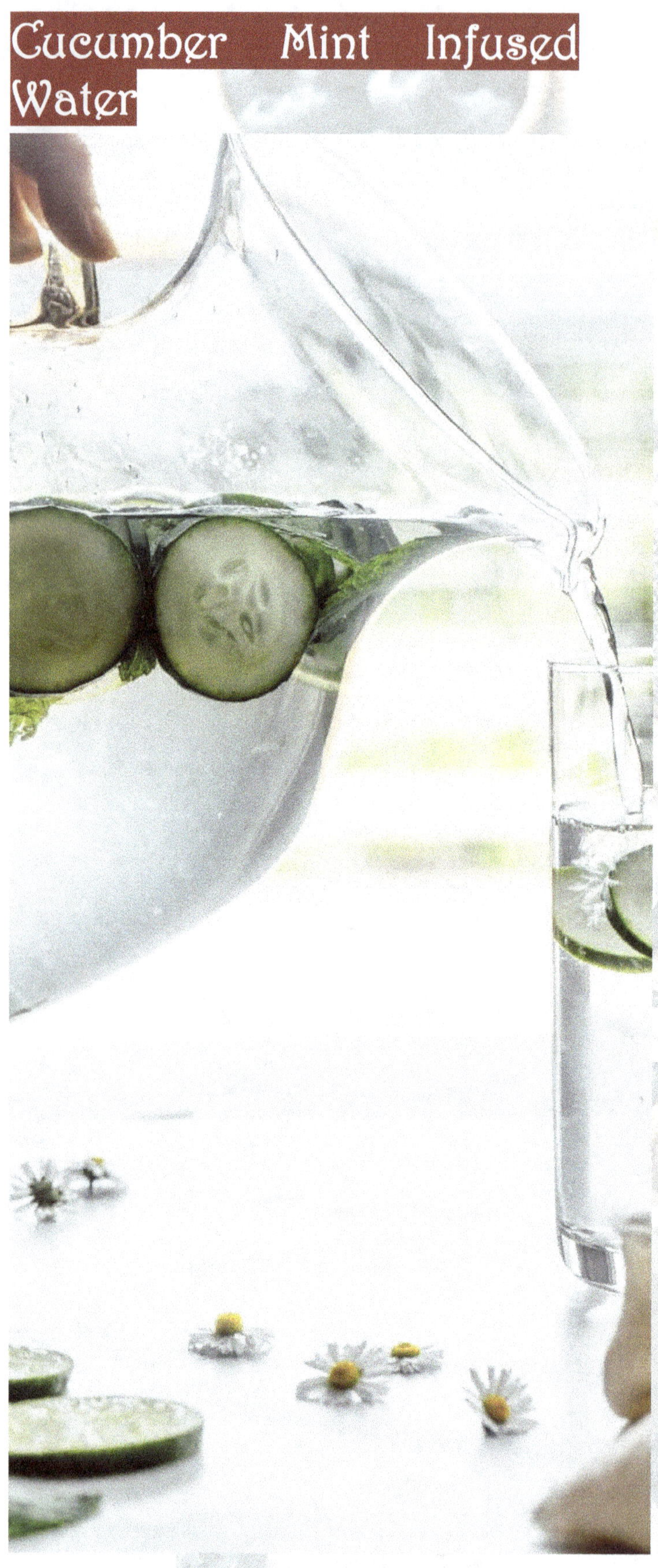

- **Preparation Time:** 10 minutes
- **Cooking Time:** None
- **Serving:** 4

Ingredients:

- 1 cucumber, thinly sliced
- 1/4 cup fresh mint leaves
- 8 cups water & Ice cubes (optional)

Procedure:

1. In a large pitcher, combine the cucumber slices and mint leaves.
2. Fill the pitcher with water and stir gently.
3. Refrigerate for at least 1 hour to allow the flavors to infuse.
4. Add ice cubes before serving if desired.
5. Serve cold and enjoy!

Nutritional Values (per serving):

- Calories: 0
- Protein: 0g
- Carbohydrates: 0g
- Fiber: 0g
- Sugars: 0g
- Fat: 0g
- Saturated Fat: 0g
- Sodium: 0mg

Health Benefits:

- **Hydration:** Helps maintain proper hydration levels.
- **Refreshing and Detoxifying:** Cucumber and mint provide a refreshing taste and support detoxification.

Green Tea Smoothie

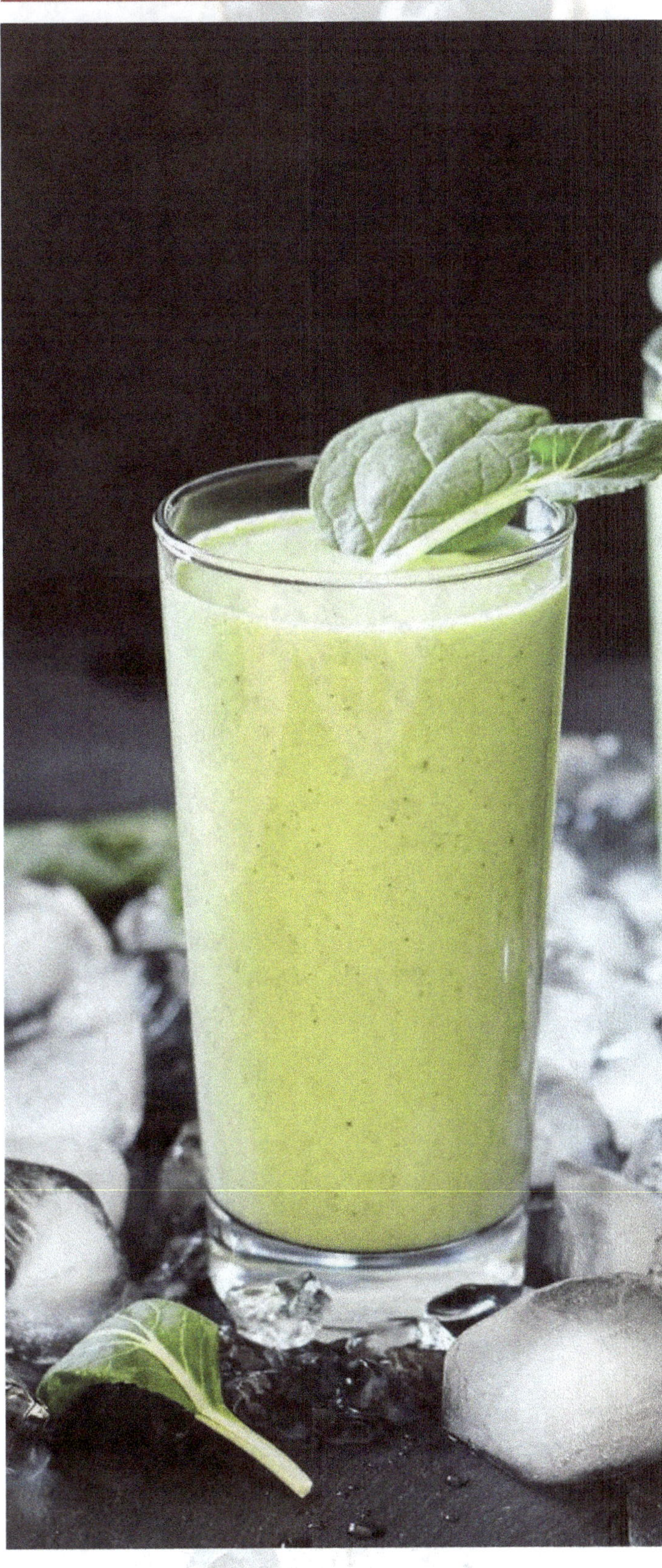

- **Preparation Time:** 10 minutes
- **Cooking Time:** None
- **Serving:** 2

Ingredients:

- 1 cup unsweetened green tea, cooled
- 1 cup spinach
- 1/2 cup Greek yogurt (plain, non-fat)
- 1/2 cup frozen mango chunks
- 1/2 banana
- 1 tablespoon chia seeds
- 1 teaspoon honey or a few drops of stevia (optional)

Procedure:

1. Brew green tea and let it cool.
2. In a blender, combine cooled green tea, spinach, Greek yogurt, frozen mango chunks, banana, chia seeds, and honey (or stevia).
3. Blend until smooth and creamy.
4. Pour into glasses and serve immediately.
5. Enjoy!

Nutritional Values (per serving):

- Calories: 150
- Protein: 7g
- Carbohydrates: 25g
- Fiber: 5g
- Sugars: 15g (natural sugars from fruit)
- Fat: 3g
- Saturated Fat: 1g
- Sodium: 40mg

Health Benefits:

- **Antioxidants:** Green tea and spinach are rich in antioxidants that help reduce inflammation.

- **High Fiber:** Chia seeds and fruits provide fiber, aiding in blood sugar control and digestion.

- **Protein-Packed:** Greek yogurt adds protein, promoting muscle maintenance and satiety.

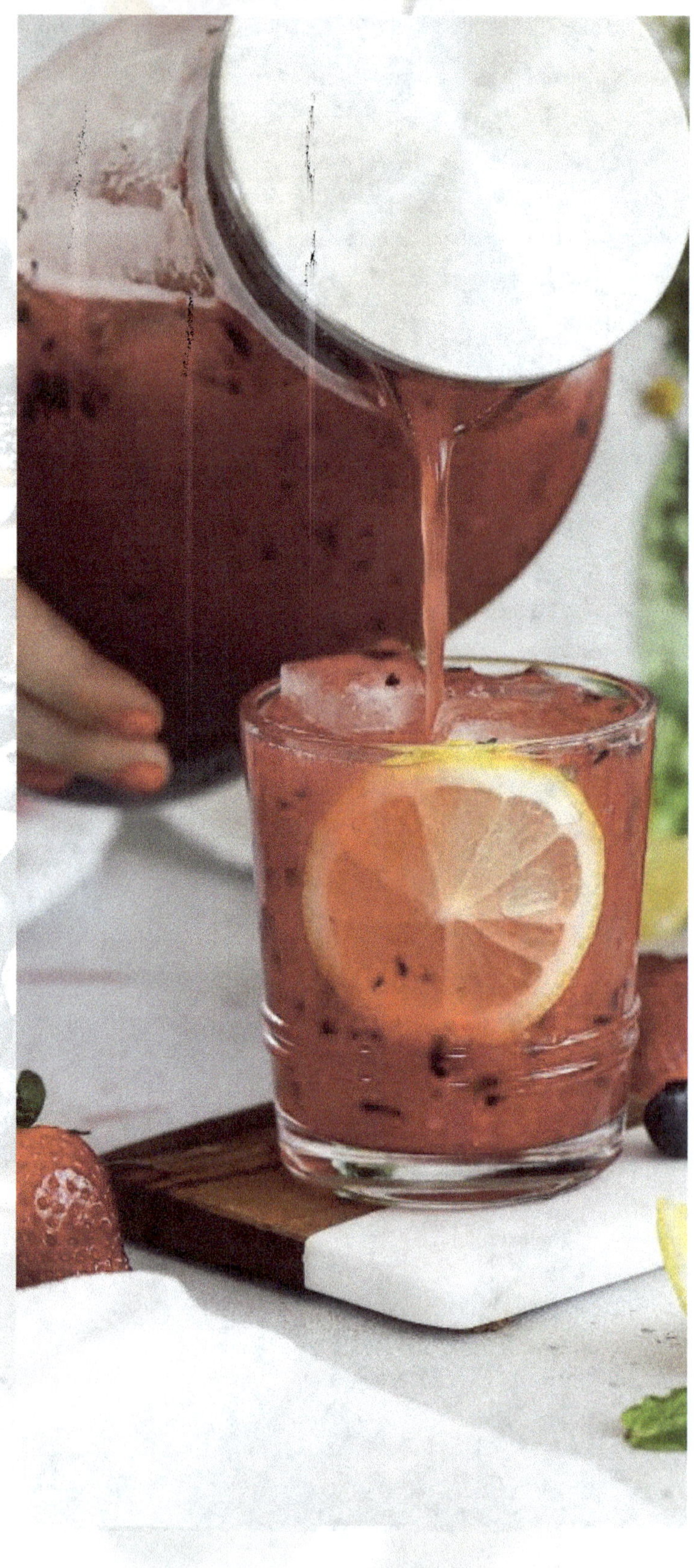

- **Preparation Time:** 10 minutes
- **Cooking Time:** None
- **Serving:** 4

Ingredients:

- 1 cup mixed berries (strawberries, blueberries, raspberries)
- 1/2 cup fresh lemon juice (about 3 lemons)
- 4 cups water
- 2 tablespoons honey or a few drops of stevia
- Ice cubes (optional)
- Lemon slices and fresh mint for garnish (optional)

Procedure:

1. In a blender, combine mixed berries, fresh lemon juice, water, and honey (or stevia). Blend until smooth.
2. Strain the mixture through a fine mesh sieve into a pitcher to remove seeds and pulp.
3. Refrigerate for at least 1 hour to chill.
4. Add ice cubes before serving if desired.
5. Garnish with lemon slices and fresh mint if desired.
6. Serve cold and enjoy!

Nutritional Values (per serving):

- Calories: 40
- Protein: 1g
- Carbohydrates: 10g
- Fiber: 2g
- Sugars: 8g (from berries and honey)
- Fat: 0g
- Saturated Fat: 0g
- Sodium: 5mg

Health Benefits:

- **Antioxidants:** Berries are rich in antioxidants that support overall health and reduce inflammation.
- **Low Glycemic Index:** Helps maintain stable blood sugar levels.
- **Hydration:** Provides a refreshing and hydrating beverage option.

Ginger Turmeric Tea

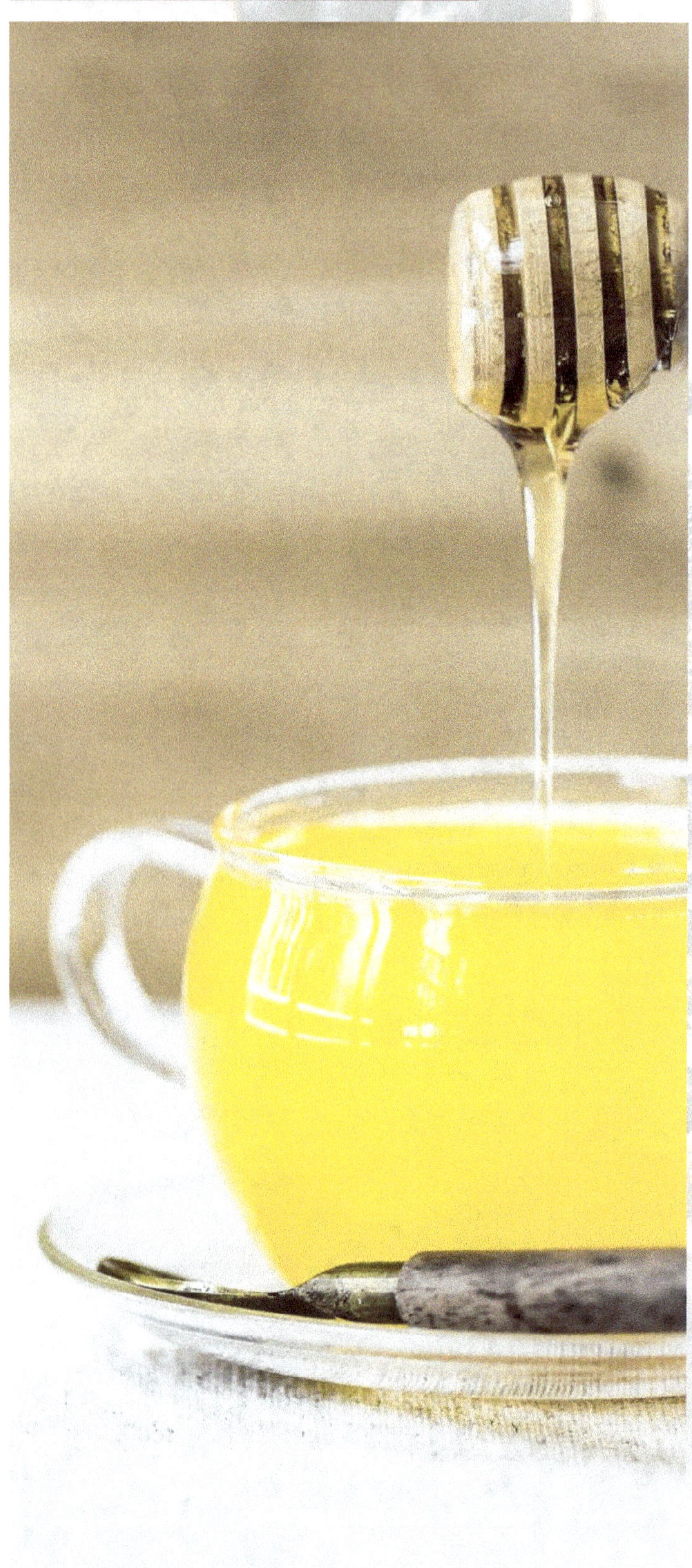

- **Preparation Time:** 10 minutes
- **Cooking Time:** 10 minutes
- **Serving:** 2

Ingredients:

- 2 cups water
- 1-inch piece fresh ginger, peeled and sliced
- 1 teaspoon ground turmeric or 1-inch piece fresh turmeric, peeled and sliced
- 1 tablespoon honey or a few drops of stevia
- 1 tablespoon lemon juice
- Black pepper (a pinch)

Procedure:

1. In a small pot, bring water to a boil.
2. Add sliced ginger and turmeric to the boiling water. Reduce heat and simmer for 10 minutes.
3. Strain the tea into cups to remove the ginger and turmeric slices.
4. Stir in honey (or stevia), lemon juice, and a pinch of black pepper.
5. Serve hot and enjoy!

Nutritional Values (per serving):

- Calories: 20
- Protein: 0g
- Carbohydrates: 5g
- Fiber: 0g
- Sugars: 4g (from honey)
- Fat: 0g
- Saturated Fat: 0g
- Sodium: 0mg

Health Benefits:

- **Anti-Inflammatory:** Ginger and turmeric are known for their anti-inflammatory properties.

- **Digestive Health:** Ginger aids in digestion and can help relieve nausea.

- **Immune Support:** Turmeric and ginger support the immune system and overall health.

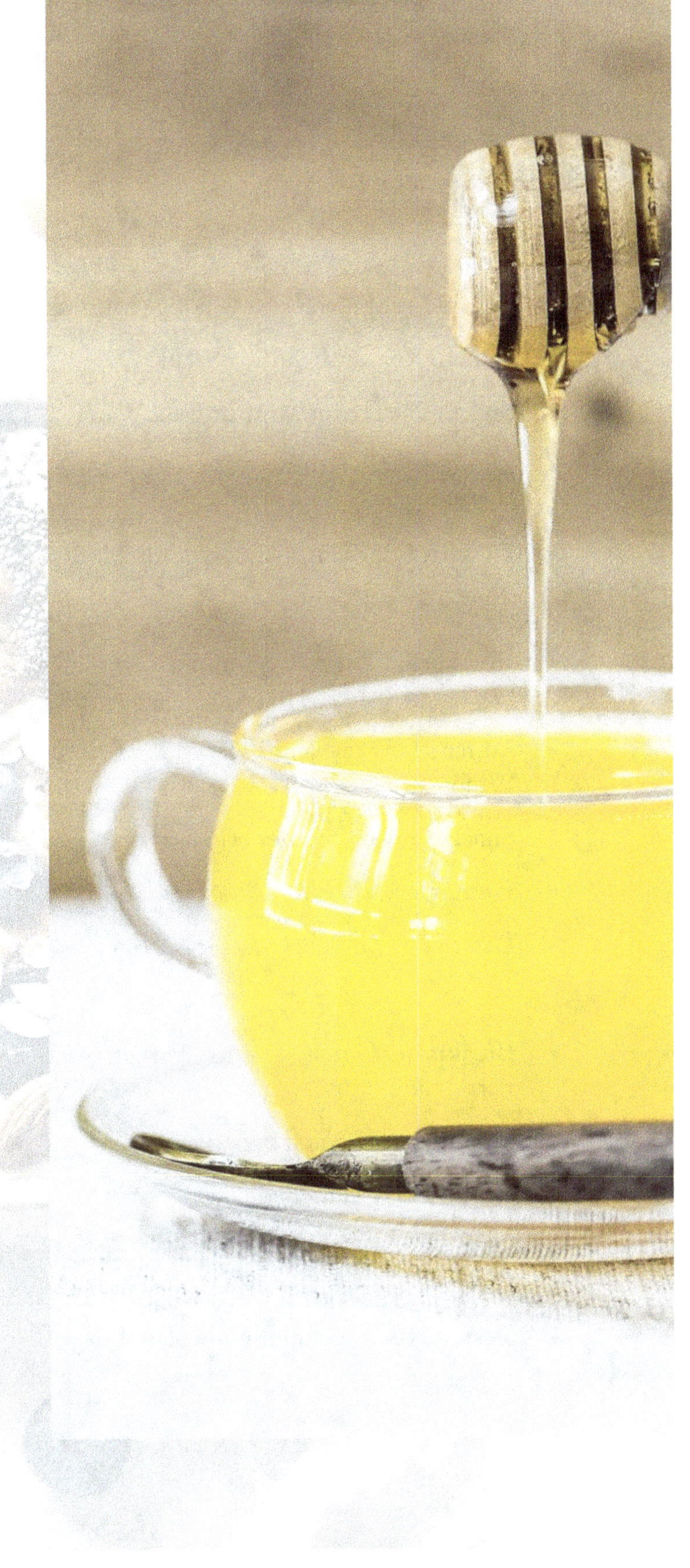

Diabetic-Friendly 4 week Meal Plan

1-Week Meal Plan (Week 1)

Day 1

- **Breakfast:** Spinach and Feta Egg Muffins
- **Lunch:** Kale and Quinoa Salad
- **Snack:** Cucumber Mint Infused Water
- **Dinner:** Herb-Crusted Cod with Roasted Veggies
- **Dessert:** Dark Chocolate Avocado Mousse

Day 2

- **Breakfast:** Blueberry Almond Overnight Oats
- **Lunch:** Turkey and Avocado Lettuce Wraps
- **Snack:** Ginger Turmeric Tea
- **Dinner:** Slow Cooker Beef Stew
- **Dessert:** Sugar-Free Cheesecake Bites

Day 3

- **Breakfast:** Greek Yogurt Parfait with Berries and Nuts
- **Lunch:** Spinach and Strawberry Salad
- **Snack:** Berry Lemonade
- **Dinner:** Grilled Chicken and Veggie Wrap
- **Dessert:** Peanut Butter Chocolate Bites

Day 4

- **Breakfast:** Peanut Butter Banana Smoothie
- **Lunch:** Mixed Greens with Lemon Vinaigrette
- **Snack:** Cucumber and Tomato Salad with Feta
- **Dinner:** Vegetable and Tofu Stir-Fry
- **Dessert:** Baked Apples with Cinnamon

Day 5

- **Breakfast:** Chia Seed Pudding with Mango
- **Lunch:** Lentil and Spinach Soup
- **Snack:** Green Tea Smoothie
- **Dinner:** Baked Lemon Herb Salmon
- **Dessert:** Pumpkin Spice Mug Cake

Day 6

- **Breakfast:** Quinoa and Black Bean Salad
- **Lunch:** Butternut Squash and Apple Soup
- **Snack:** Roasted Beet and Goat Cheese Salad
- **Dinner:** Chicken and Broccoli Stir-Fry
- **Dessert:** Coconut Macaroons

Day 7

- **Breakfast:** Berry Lemonade
- **Lunch:** Creamy Cauliflower Soup
- **Snack:** Cucumber Mint Infused Water
- **Dinner:** Grilled Pork Chops with Apple Slaw
- **Dessert:** Dark Chocolate Avocado Mousse

1-Week Meal Plan (Week 2)

Day 1

- **Breakfast:** Veggie-Packed Breakfast Burrito
- **Lunch:** Greek Yogurt Parfait with Berries and Nuts
- **Snack:** Berry Chia Pudding
- **Dinner:** Turkey Meatballs with Zucchini Noodles
- **Dessert:** Baked Apples with Cinnamon

Day 2

- **Breakfast:** Chia Seed Pudding with Mango
- **Lunch:** Quinoa and Black Bean Salad
- **Snack:** Cucumber Mint Infused Water
- **Dinner:** Grilled Chicken and Veggie Wrap
- **Dessert:** Sugar-Free Cheesecake Bites

Day 3

- **Breakfast:** Peanut Butter Banana Smoothie
- **Lunch:** Spinach and Strawberry Salad
- **Snack:** Ginger Turmeric Tea
- **Dinner:** Baked Lemon Herb Salmon
- **Dessert:** Pumpkin Spice Mug Cake

Day 4

- **Breakfast:** Dark Chocolate Avocado Mousse
- **Lunch:** Lentil and Spinach Soup
- **Snack:** Green Tea Smoothie
- **Dinner:** Chicken and Broccoli Stir-Fry
- **Dessert:** Coconut Macaroons

Day 5

- **Breakfast:** Blueberry Almond Overnight Oats
- **Lunch:** Mixed Greens with Lemon Vinaigrette
- **Snack:** Berry Lemonade
- **Dinner:** Herb-Crusted Cod with Roasted Veggies
- **Dessert:** Peanut Butter Chocolate Bites

Day 6

- **Breakfast:** Greek Yogurt Parfait with Berries and Nuts
- **Lunch:** Butternut Squash and Apple Soup
- **Snack:** Cucumber and Tomato Salad with Feta
- **Dinner:** Slow Cooker Beef Stew
- **Dessert:** Dark Chocolate Avocado Mousse

Day 7

- **Breakfast:** Spinach and Feta Egg Muffins
- **Lunch:** Creamy Cauliflower Soup
- **Snack:** Cucumber Mint Infused Water
- **Dinner:** Shrimp and Asparagus Stir-Fry
- **Dessert:** Sugar-Free Cheesecake Bites

1-Week Meal Plan (Week 3)

Day 1

- **Breakfast:** Spinach and Feta Egg Muffins
- **Lunch:** Mixed Greens with Lemon Vinaigrette
- **Snack:** Cucumber Mint Infused Water
- **Dinner:** Herb-Crusted Cod with Roasted Veggies
- **Dessert:** Dark Chocolate Avocado Mousse

Day 2

- **Breakfast:** Blueberry Almond Overnight Oats
- **Lunch:** Lentil and Spinach Soup
- **Snack:** Green Tea Smoothie
- **Dinner:** Grilled Chicken and Veggie Wrap
- **Dessert:** Sugar-Free Cheesecake Bites

Day 3

- **Breakfast:** Greek Yogurt Parfait with Berries and Nuts
- **Lunch:** Spinach and Strawberry Salad
- **Snack:** Berry Lemonade
- **Dinner:** Slow Cooker Beef Stew
- **Dessert:** Peanut Butter Chocolate Bites

Day 4

- **Breakfast:** Peanut Butter Banana Smoothie
- **Lunch:** Cucumber and Tomato Salad with Feta
- **Snack:** Ginger Turmeric Tea
- **Dinner:** Baked Lemon Herb Salmon
- **Dessert:** Baked Apples with Cinnamon

Day 5

- **Breakfast:** Chia Seed Pudding with Mango
- **Lunch:** Quinoa and Black Bean Salad
- **Snack:** Cucumber Mint Infused Water
- **Dinner:** Chicken and Broccoli Stir-Fry
- **Dessert:** Coconut Macaroons

Day 6

- **Breakfast:** Dark Chocolate Avocado Mousse
- **Lunch:** Butternut Squash and Apple Soup
- **Snack:** Berry Chia Pudding
- **Dinner:** Vegetable and Tofu Stir-Fry
- **Dessert:** Pumpkin Spice Mug Cake

Day 7

- **Breakfast:** Greek Yogurt Parfait with Berries and Nuts
- **Lunch:** Kale and Quinoa Salad
- **Snack:** Cucumber Mint Infused Water
- **Dinner:** Shrimp and Asparagus Stir-Fry
- **Dessert:** Sugar-Free Cheesecake Bites

Day 1

- **Breakfast:** Blueberry Almond Overnight Oats
- **Lunch:** Mixed Greens with Lemon Vinaigrette
- **Snack:** Cucumber Mint Infused Water
- **Dinner:** Herb-Crusted Cod with Roasted Veggies
- **Dessert:** Sugar-Free Cheesecake Bites

Day 2

- **Breakfast:** Greek Yogurt Parfait with Berries and Nuts
- **Lunch:** Lentil and Spinach Soup
- **Snack:** Green Tea Smoothie
- **Dinner:** Chicken and Broccoli Stir-Fry
- **Dessert:** Dark Chocolate Avocado Mousse

Day 3

- **Breakfast:** Peanut Butter Banana Smoothie
- **Lunch:** Cucumber and Tomato Salad with Feta
- **Snack:** Berry Lemonade
- **Dinner:** Baked Lemon Herb Salmon
- **Dessert:** Pumpkin Spice Mug Cake

Day 4

- **Breakfast:** Spinach and Feta Egg Muffins
- **Lunch:** Kale and Quinoa Salad
- **Snack:** Ginger Turmeric Tea
- **Dinner:** Slow Cooker Beef Stew
- **Dessert:** Peanut Butter Chocolate Bites

Day 5

- **Breakfast:** Chia Seed Pudding with Mango
- **Lunch:** Spinach and Strawberry Salad
- **Snack:** Cucumber Mint Infused Water
- **Dinner:** Grilled Chicken and Veggie Wrap
- **Dessert:** Baked Apples with Cinnamon

Day 6

- **Breakfast:** Dark Chocolate Avocado Mousse
- **Lunch:** Butternut Squash and Apple Soup
- **Snack:** Berry Chia Pudding
- **Dinner:** Vegetable and Tofu Stir-Fry
- **Dessert:** Coconut Macaroons

Day 7

- **Breakfast:** Greek Yogurt Parfait with Berries and Nuts
- **Lunch:** Quinoa and Black Bean Salad
- **Snack:** Cucumber Mint Infused Water
- **Dinner:** Shrimp and Asparagus Stir-Fry
- **Dessert:** Sugar-Free Cheesecake Bites

Shopping List for "Diabetic Cookbook Made Simple for Seniors

Produce

- Spinach (fresh and frozen)
- Blueberries
- Kale
- Quinoa
- Cucumber
- Mint Leaves
- Zucchini
- Cherry Tomatoes
- Red Onion
- Bell Peppers (variety)
- Carrots
- Strawberries
- Avocado
- Mixed Greens (arugula, spinach, lettuce)
- Beets
- Apples
- Bananas
- Mango
- Butternut Squash
- Broccoli
- Cauliflower
- Garlic
- Ginger
- Lemons
- Limes
- Asparagus
- Snap Peas
- Baby Carrots
- Celery
- Fresh Parsley
- Fresh Dill
- Fresh Basil
- Fresh Thyme
- Fresh Cilantro
- Fresh Chives

Protein

- Chicken Breasts (boneless, skinless)
- Turkey Breasts
- Lean Beef Stew Meat
- Cod Fillets
- Tofu (firm)
- Greek Yogurt (plain, non-fat)
- Eggs
- Shrimp (peeled, deveined)
- Ricotta Cheese (part-skim)
- Ground Turkey

Dairy

- Unsweetened Almond Milk
- Part-Skim Mozzarella Cheese
- Parmesan Cheese
- Feta Cheese
- Goat Cheese

Pantry Staples

- Olive Oil
- Coconut Oil
- Apple Cider Vinegar
- Balsamic Vinegar
- Red Wine Vinegar
- Dijon Mustard
- Honey or Stevia
- Unsweetened Cocoa Powder
- Vanilla Extract
- Rolled Oats
- Almond Flour
- Coconut Flour
- Chia Seeds
- Sunflower Seeds
- Dried Cranberries (unsweetened)
- Walnuts
- Dark Chocolate Chips (optional)
- Natural Peanut Butter (no added sugar)
- Low-Sodium Soy Sauce

- Low-Sodium Chicken Broth
- Low-Sodium Beef Broth
- Low-Sodium Vegetable Broth
- Diced Tomatoes (canned)
- Low-Sodium Marinara Sauce
- Whole Wheat Tortillas

Spices and Seasonings

- Black Pepper
- Salt
- Ground Turmeric
- Ground Cinnamon
- Ground Nutmeg
- Ground Cumin
- Ground Coriander
- Dried Thyme
- Dried Basil
- Dried Oregano
- Paprika
- Red Pepper Flakes
- Garlic Powder
- Onion Powder
- Ground Ginger
- Italian Seasoning

Beverages

- Green Tea (bags or loose leaf)
- Herbal Tea (ginger, mint, turmeric)

This list ensures that all necessary ingredients for the specified recipes are included.

Conclusion

Congratulations, you've reached the end of *Diabetic Cookbook Made Simple for Seniors*! But don't worry, this isn't goodbye—it's just the beginning of a delicious and healthier chapter in your life.

Remember when managing diabetes felt like a daunting task? With the help of these easy and tasty recipes, you've transformed your kitchen into a culinary powerhouse, dishing out meals that are as delightful as they are nutritious. Gone are the days of bland, uninspired dishes; instead, you're now a master of flavors, balancing carbs, proteins, and healthy fats like a pro.

Think back to the first time you tried the Baked Lemon Herb Salmon or the Pumpkin Spice Mug Cake. Those were just the appetizers in your journey toward culinary excellence and diabetes management. Each recipe was designed to keep your blood sugar levels steady without sacrificing taste or enjoyment. And let's not forget those refreshing beverages like the Ginger Turmeric Tea—who knew managing diabetes could be so refreshing?

Now, you're armed with a repertoire of meals that not only support your health but also bring joy to your dining table. You've learned that eating well doesn't mean giving up the foods you love; it's about finding creative ways to make them work for you.

As you continue on this journey, remember to experiment and have fun. Mix and match ingredients, try new spices, and don't be afraid to make these recipes your own. After all, the kitchen is your playground.

So, here's to you and your newfound culinary skills! Keep cooking, keep experimenting, and most importantly, keep enjoying every bite. Because managing diabetes isn't just about making healthier choices—it's about savoring them too. Bon appétit!

www.ingramcontent.com/pod-product-compliance
Lightning Source LLC
Chambersburg PA
CBHW081557250726
48653CB00009B/3466